# From Sickness To Health

## by
## Fruitarianna

To contact the author write to Fruitarianna at hello@fruitarianna.com.
Available for purchase in paperback and e-book formats at SweetVeganNature.com/shop.
Cover, design and book editing by Anna Chmielewska.
Special thanks to Fiona Arakelian for proofreading.

*He who takes medicine*
*and neglects the diet*
*wastes the skill*
*of his doctors*

*—Chinese Proverb*

# Acknowledgments

Most of the science explained in this book I learned from lectures by Dr. Joel Robbins, who teaches the simple truth about the origins of disease and body self-healing capabilities. For months I've been studying it and passing forward what I learnt that works and together with over 2 years of research, practice and couching others I came up with the content for this book. I am also grateful for the teachings by Dr. T. Colin Campbell, Arnold N. Kauffman, Dr. Dough Graham and his wife, Professor Rozalind Graham and Gary Yourofsky. Thank you all for living what you are teaching and showing the way to a sickness-free, vibrant living.

# About the content

The book consists of three sections. In the first part, the **Introduction**, you get to know my story and a bit of my background. Next is the **Manual** part where you will learn about the origins of disease and how to stay healthy by following the nature's clues. Lastly, you there are **Further readings** with complimentary topics. Feel free if to skip it if they do not resonate with you. In my mind, this book wouldn't be complete without them.

If you have any questions please do not hesitate to write to me at hello@fruitarianna.com.

With all my love,
I dedicate this book to my mom.
You are constantly opening my heart.
I love you very much!

# Index

Introduction     8

## The Manual     13

## Chapter 1: Basics     13

Why do we get sick?     14
Compounds of disease     14
The source behind healing     15

## Chapter 2: Junk food vs. real food     16

Why do we eat?     16
What are toxins?     22

## Chapter 3: Toxins and stimulants     26

How do we compensate the lack of energy?     27

## Chapter 4: Inorganic vs. organic     31

Vitamins and supplements—organic vs. synthetic     32
The hierarchy of food processing     33

## Chapter 5: Disease and the healing process     34

About pH     34
How do we get sick?     35
The disease process     38
The processed foods era     48
The healing crisis     50
Incurable diseases     52
Weight loss game     53
How long does it take to get healthy?     53

# Further readings 55

It's important how you start 56
Appetite and satisfaction 56
Eating enough for weight loss 58

**Transition diet** 60
Smoothies 60
Salad and dressings 61
Main dishes 62
Desserts 69

Herbs, spices and seaweed 66
Fasting 67
About digestion 69
Social situations 72
Relationship with food 73
Shortly about bulimia 73
Food combinations 75
Alkaline foods 77

**About veganism** 78

# Recommended 84

# Introduction

## About the author

### My name is Anna and this a story of Fruitarianna[1]

In my early 20's I was obsessed with training for performance when I discovered the protein diet, that supposed to help me to get stronger and ripen (to reduce the fat in my body). For someone who gets her education about nutrition from women's magazines and mainstream medical "know-how," meat-based diet sounded convincing enough to change my whole diet.

The protein-based diet consists of meat, fish, low-fat dairy, cooked or raw, and nothing else. I ate boiled eggs for breakfast, baked chicken or turkey breast for lunch, steamed fish for dinner and tuna with low-fat cottage cheese as my last meal. I also made sure to drink lots and lots of water as advised, and I had to shower 4-5 times a day, as this lifestyle and diet made me sweat excessively. Thank god for the shower in the office!

My routine was simple. I woke up at 5:30am for a morning run 1-hour gym class at 7am before work, to return 9 hours later for a weight-lifting session. After that I often would go back to work for a couple more hours, filling the role of a responsible manager. It was one of the most intensive periods in my life. I was giving my best in the gym, at the office and to my clients.

One morning, about 6 months after the diet change, I woke up and I realized I couldn't stand up. I collapsed and fell asleep. Next 10 days I spent in bed completely spaced out and barely able to move. My systems were down for about a month after my body rebelled—I had no choice but to rest. So I was sleeping, drinking water only and being so fed up with meat that even my mom's famous chicken soup couldn't win my affection at that time. I remember eating few apples and some bananas and I can't forget the delicious taste of blueberries my brother brought me once! Other than that I was just resting and fasting.

From that point, I couldn't eat meat anymore. It wasn't a conscious choice though, it just happened that I stopped buying and preparing any meat for myself. Cooked vegetarian

---

[1] *Fruitarianna* is a comic character, Anna's alter ego. In her comic Fruitarianna talks about nutrition and health-related topics in a simple, fun and colorful way. Follow her journey as she discovers more facts and busts some myths at fruitarianna.com.

diet was my thing and I really enjoyed exploring new ways of baking tarts, quiches, pates and veggie stews.

I gave up the gym and I slowed down at work. In a short time I started gaining weight, and then I remembered—I used to be a bulimic, what a fantastic way out! Why not to get back to that practice, I thought. It's interesting how easy it is to hide bulimia from everybody. I "learned" bulimia when I was still in high school. Now, 14 years later, I can say—I'm free! I conquered it when I discovered the abundant way of eating juicy fruits and fresh vegetables, leafy greens and some nuts and seeds. This is what I thrive on now! But it didn't change within one day, not yet at least.

At the age of 29 I moved to Amsterdam to take a break in my career, and after a year and a half I moved to London, where I got back to being a manager again. Here, when I reached the top of my weight, being over 20 kg from where I feel comfortable at, I finally discovered the solution to rewrite my never-ending weight-gaining story.

I learned about a plant-based diet—raw, unspoiled, fresh and life-giving source of nutrients. As I was watching people's countless testimonials on YouTube I noticed what they all had in common—aside from conquering health issues and incurable diseases such as diabetes, Lyme disease or cancer—they had lost weight, some had beaten bulimia. They all looked genuinely happy and so vibrant! Watching 60-, 70- year-old women being vegan half their lives and looking better than most 40-year-old, I knew who I need to follow and seek advice from to preserve my youth and be healthy and fit again.

I watched and read every article about nutrition, plant-source of protein and glucose, our basic fuel, human body's bio-chemistry and anatomy, and I was mesmerized with the simplicity of our body's mechanics. I was wandering, why we haven't been taught that at school? The message was simple and I was about to dive deep to understand it all.

I knew already the best way to become an expert in a topic is by being able to explain it to others. I got involved in coaching groups and individuals when I was living in United States, working side-by-side Arnold Kauffman at his wonderful Arnold's Way Healing Center and Vegan Café. After countless hours of answering questions I decided to put all I learnt in writing. That's how this book came to life. I leave you with this book in your hands to help you too understand that there's no mystery in creating health, neither to creating sickness. Please share this message with all everyone for sickness-free world!

# Come for a journey

In spite of my first career choice, I always was a teacher, or better still—a story teller, although it wasn't so clear to me until the last few years. People often tell me that they love the way I tell the stories and I hope you will enjoy this one. I'm excited and grateful to have the opportunity every time there's an attentive listener. To hear that I helped somebody to gain health or to save someone's life is precious to me!

I wish I could tell you a story the way I do, face to face, with passion, celebrating those moments of eureka when you are starting to understand it all too—It's all so simple! I wish I could tell you the story that will open your eyes to the possibility that humanity made a wrong turn in the past, choosing to dominate the world for the doom of our health and animals welfare. I wish I could tell you that your eating habits are good and all you need is to buy that new super-duper supplement or that there is a super food remedy for everything. Or, just like your doctors advice—take four of those red pills and all your health problems will be gone.

Instead, I want to tell you I love you and I care for you. Instead, I want to share a story of how your body works that may not be pretty sometimes but hey, who says the truth has to be? I want to take you on a journey so you can see for yourself whether what I'm saying makes any sense to you. But don't take me for an authority, I may be all wrong! Instead, use your critical thinking and, if you feel that what I'm suggesting sounds good to you, try it! Know that everyone has an opinion and it's impossible to discuss it all, as it's impossible to see the effects of our dietary choices immediately, sometimes it takes all your life! But there will always be somebody who will tell you whatever you want to hear, just so you buy another product or another miraculous health-giving pill.

Remember, only you are responsible for your health, so please, use your common sense on this journey. Are you ready to follow me down into the rabbit hole? I promise that there's a light at the end of the tunnel.

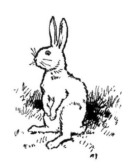

*I wish you, your family, friends and pets*
*a lifetime of good health and happiness!*

*—Fruitarianna*

# About medical healthcare

The hospital industry is the fifth largest industry in the United States. Despite this already in 1985 the American Medical Association and the World Health Organization both stated, that America has the worst epidemic of chronic, degenerative disease that mankind has ever known. We are talking about cancer, arthritis, diabetes and heart disease.

Here's what I see—a patient goes to a doctor and he lists his symptoms. Five days and $5,000 later the test results are back. The doctor lines up the test results with the symptoms given and he comes up with the name of disease. Now, the patient feels relief, since the doctor knows the name of disease he must know how to treat it, right? Meanwhile, in the medical school future MD's learn that 95% of the disease's cause known today is **UNKNOWN**!

So the question is this: how can we treat something if we don't know what causes it? And yet, the doctors open their medical bible and they come up with the "treatment of the day," based on the tests results, that are either a drug, therapy or surgery procedure. But again, how can we treat something if we don't know what causes it?

Think about that, if you have a headache, and you go to a doctor, he'll prescribe you an aspirin. Does that mean you have an aspirin deficiency? I've never heard of that! I've never heard of a **vitamin-pill deficiency** causing a disease, although I've heard of **vitamin deficiencies** causing a disease.

*FACT:* Where do those **vitamin deficiencies** come from? From **not eating the foods** that have the **vitamins** in them!

11

# The principle we operate by

In general, the medical doctors and natural healing practitioners are operating by the same principal when it comes to treating patients. What is this principal?

> Providing a **symptomatic relief** <u>without</u> the patient having to <u>change</u> whatever they were doing wrong that <u>caused the problem</u> in the first place.

The cause and effect in this case would be that if you violate the law of this body there is a price to be paid, and there's no around it. It's like saying:

*"Give me the pill to sober me up but please, let me keep drinking."*

Remember this, everybody has a different opinion and you will always find someone who will tell you whatever it is you want to hear. One will tell you there's no such thing as a junk food; the other will tell you fruit is the only food you should eat. It is because the laws that govern this universe do not always pay right now. The consequences aren't always felt immediately. Sometimes it takes a lifetime.

Reading this book will shine a light on your understanding of the simplicity of how your body works, showing you what to do to improve your health. Learn how to enable your body's healing capabilities to reverse disease you've been medicating without hope of getting better. Understand and apply the simple steps I'm showing you here and you will get in charge of your future in no time, without much effort.

 *Please know that I do not take responsibility for the results you will get, as you and only you are responsible for your actions and health. Know that what I share here worked for me and anybody I worked with. If you seek advice or something is unclear, please contact me for support to get better results. I'd be happy to help you on your journey to health.*

# The Manual

# Chapter 1: Basics

# Why do we get sick?

I believe that there are only two reasons why we get sick. First is **ignorance**, second - **laziness**. So you honestly didn't know that eating fatty foods makes you fat? And now that you finally know, how about applying it? Tough, isn't it?

It can be challenging to maintain health after the age of 30, when you don't give your body what it calls for and you used so much of your reserves already. If you numb yourself with processed foods, composed of dead products that slowly add to your heart and digestion problems, you create immobility and bring suffering to your body. How about feeling energized, mindful and looking young and vibrant instead?

If I can help you understand how the food plays the part in our health, whether in the disease or in the healing process, then you will realize that there's no mystery to it and you too can gain all the powers I'm talking about.

# Compounds of disease

Disease is an unnatural state as a result of body's toxication, lack of rest and nutrients. The body doesn't know how to get sick, but it has its own ways to prevent it from dying, that can sometimes lead to a serious condition. Before we learn how it comes to that, let's learn about our body's healing capabilities.

# The Source Behind Healing

Have you noticed that all life designed and created by nature needs no supervision to grow, multiply and give fruit (or babies), when in the right environment? No animal in nature gets sick and needs to take pills and days off, so would it be fair to assume that even such complex system as human body is governed by the same *innate intelligence* that is supporting all life processes?

If at conception this alive cell that soon is about to be a human being doesn't need a doctor to assist, why should we struggle with our health later on? What if we were equipped with an intelligent system that will always try to get healthy, regardless of the cost? Don't our wounds heal if we let them? As long as we stay away from the process, sooner or later our broken bones grow back together and our tissues close and wounds heal, right? So shouldn't it be the same case with other conditions like heart or colon disease?

Know that the body doesn't know how to get sick, it only knows how to get healthy. It is only when we interfere, we get in trouble.

Let me ask you this—do you remember having a hangover after poisoning yourself with alcohol during the party the night before? You knew exactly how it's going to end but you didn't stop drinking, did you? This is what I mean when I say we are getting sick because of our ignorance or laziness. But the innate intelligence strives to keep the body alive regardless of the cost. Soon, you will understand what it means to your health as we progress.

# Chapter 2: Junk food vs. real food

It looks like everyone agrees that McDonald's, pizza, chips, cotton candy or microwave-ready meals are junk foods. Those foods are often high in sugar, fats, salt and unpronounceable chemicals, making it a calorie-dense meal that is of little nutritional value. These so-called "comfort foods" lack vitamins, minerals and water, without which we can't be healthy. This may not mean much to you yet so, in order to understand the difference, and what happens inside the body when we eat the food, we need to learn first what the real food is and what its role is.

# Why do we eat?

It's simple—we eat to live. We eat because we need glucose to run on; protein—to build our body; fats—to produce hormones; vitamins and minerals—to run it all effectively and we need water to keep us hydrated and to run any process inside our body. If a food consists of those six elements only, it is considered to be **real food** for humans.

> The **real food** has it all in one package—the perfect 6:
> glucose • protein • fatty acids • minerals • vitamins • water

# 1.  Glucose

Cars run on gas, humans run on glucose. It's as simple as that, and that is **the main reason for us to eat the food**. Just like you choose carefully the right fuel for your car, you may think twice next time you feel tired, running on reserve. Coffee has only as much glucose as you will put sugar in it, the rest is a simply blood-raising drug but a banana is just 90% carbohydrates!

We all have sweet tooth to recognize what's poison and what's the real food—this is how we were designed. If only we didn't spoil our taste buds with spices and strong-tasting foods we would have no doubts about it. Kids know so!

> *Have you ever heard: "Don't eat sweets before dinner, you're going to spoil your appetite!"? Well, I eat sweets for my breakfast and for dinner because I want to spoil my appetite! I eat so much sweet fruit until I'm not hungry anymore. Then I go back to work or I go out and play. Because my meals are simple and easy to digest I don't need any siesta! Energized I'm up and ready to go.*

# 2.  Protein

Protein is the building structure of the body. A growing child will need up to 20% of protein in the diet, but grown up human beings need only as much as 10%[2] of protein and no more. Research[3] has shown that eating too much protein promotes cancer growth, especially when animal protein is involved.

> *When I recall the time I was following the protein diet, eating just meat, fish, eggs and low-fat cheese, I know now that it was way more my body could handle. What do you think happened with all that extra the protein my body didn't have a use for, and wasn't able to remove quickly enough? It had to result with some abnormalities, right?*

---

[2] If you eat 2000-calorie diet you need only 200 calories coming from protein and that is the 10% of your daily nutrition needs.
[3] Read *The China Study* by Dr. T. Colin Campbell

*One day I went to a doctor complaining about breathing difficulties. When the doctor examined my x-ray she was shocked I could breathe at all having my sinuses fully stuffed with an enormous polyp. I'm still amazed the doctor wasn't able explain the origins of the tissue overgrowth, neither to link it to my diet, even after I suggested that. Doesn't it make you wonder sometimes if our doctors know better? I know now, and you should understand too, obsessing about protein is a recipe for some sort of a disaster for sure.*

Look, I'm not saying you will get polyps now, you've probably never done anything so stupid I did. But in the long run, do you know how much you eat? And where did this obsession about having enough come from? Have you ever met anybody who had a protein-deficiency disease? Of course not, there's no such thing!

Remember this for now, our bodies can't deal with the excess of protein, there's only as much space inside and so many purposes it can be used for. Eating too much protein is like bringing more bricks to a finished building site—there's no use for it and, if you leave it no choice, your body will have to come up with something creative to do with it. Once we understand we are not growing anymore and we don't need as much, especially as the body is recycling some of the proteins, it's much more important to look for the protein quality.

## What is the protein quality and where do I get the protein from?

Is the best and most bloody steak from your favorite butcher's store the best for you? I'm sure it tastes great, I won't argue with that. But into answer to what's the best for you we need to follow our digestive track and examine which proteins are effectively used in our bodies and which cause problems. **Protein quality**, from a nutrition perspective, is a term used to describe how well a protein from food matches the body's requirements and, therefore, how useful the protein is for our body. This is determined by looking at the building blocks which make up the protein called amino acids. The plant kingdom is abundant in organic (here meaning *alive*) protein and other nutrients, that are the best match for humans we should care for.

And if we are talking about the quantity—check out the kale or spinach, they have almost twice as much protein as a medium-sized steak!

*Where do I get my **protein** from?*

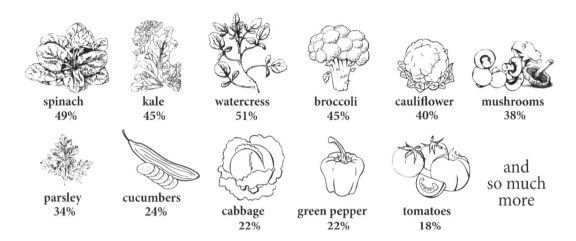

spinach 49%  kale 45%  watercress 51%  broccoli 45%  cauliflower 40%  mushrooms 38%

parsley 34%  cucumbers 24%  cabbage 22%  green pepper 22%  tomatoes 18%  and so much more

I could share a table listing all the plant sources of protein but I just want you to know that all plants, fruits, vegetables, nuts and seeds, have protein. Eat a variety of plants every day and you would never have to worry about protein in your life.

> *I recommend reading **The China Study** by T. Colin Campbell is arguably the most comprehensive study on nutrition ever done, where you can learn so much about protein and more. Campbell provides compelling evidence linking animal products to disease, including cancer, heart disease, osteoporosis, diabetes, etc.*

# 3. Fatty Acids (oils)

Fats are used for making hormones in our body, they carry vitamins around (fat-soluble vitamins such as: Vitamin A, D, E and K) and take a service part of a building structure. Thanks to fats keeping the water inside the body, our skin stays well hydrated and elastic. Recognize the difference between no-fat diet and a low-fat one, because it's a big deal, especially when you're fighting to lose weight, which I will talk about later on (read more in chapters *Weight loss game* and *Dressing Recipes*).

# 4.  Minerals

Minerals are used as part of a building structure They the work alongside vitamins to perform its individual functions.

# 5.  Vitamins

Vitamins, together with minerals serve as catalyst[4] for many processes in the human body. A catalyst is for your body to work more effectively. We do not live on vitamins, we live on glucose and protein. The vitamins and minerals help our body to use it more efficiently.

# 6.  Water

This is the last reason why we eat food for—a presence of water is necessary in every metabolic process to maintain life.

That is why we eat food, those six components right there. The real food, that is compatible with our bodies, comes as a complete package with everything we need to process it and put it to work to maintain life. It has nothing in it that will take away from life or health. And what happens for example, if you eat cooked food that is deprived of water? First, your body has to reach to its water reserves stored in the cells before it can start the digestion process. Your body will slow down, and it's not cheap either. This, like any other process in your body, requires energy that could be used to rebuild and heal your body instead.

Now, when we know what the real food is how can we be sure the food we choose is the real thing? The good news is that nature leaves us traces that are easily recognized by our inner compass. Let's see how we can find the real food easily.

---

[4] A catalyst is a substance that increases the rate of a chemical reaction without itself undergoing any permanent chemical change (source: Wikipedia).

# How to find the real food easily— the three food qualifications

Looking for the food designed for humans to eat it has to meet the following three qualifications. It has to be:

## 1. Something grown by nature

Easy to find, but since that leaves the field wide open, from nourishing bananas to poisonous belladonna, there's the second qualification to narrow the field.

## 2. Something we can pick straight from the vine and eat it without processing

Well, you could still pick belladonna from the vine and it still going to kill you. What substances would we not consider eating straight from the vine? How about grains? Can you imagine walking into the wheat field and just picking a stalk of wheat? Chewing it doesn't sound too appetizing, does it? In fact we cannot digest it in that form. We have to process it first (so it falls out from the second qualification). Following this rule we would still get in trouble picking belladonna, right? So there has to be one more condition, and it is the simplest of all as the food has to be simply yummy to the tummy, as my friend says.

## 3. Something yummy to the tummy

That means, if we sat down to a meal of just that one substance like mangoes or oranges, would we really enjoy it? Sure we would. How about an entire meal of just garlic? Doesn't sound too good, does it? If it does, you have a problem.

What is your body telling you already about that garlic and who is talking to you? That would be your taste buds. Did you know that our taste buds are our primal defensive mechanism to keep poisons out of the digestive track? We naturally have a sweet tooth, make no mistake about it. And what is it for? To identify glucose, our source of fuel and the main reason we eat food. So what's wrong with garlic? Well, when we analyze it we can see it has traces of all six elements we need in our food, but it also has something more—it has toxins.

# What are toxins?

You will learn more about toxins and irritants in next the chapter, but already we should know the basic definition, and that is:

> **Toxins** are something our body can't use, in any way, it's not designed to run on; it's the **wrong kind of fuel**. Toxic food is a junk food.

So for example, when we eat garlic our body says:

> *"Yes—I see the glucose, protein, fatty acids, vitamins, minerals and water but there's this toxin, and the cost to me to get rid of that toxin far out ways the benefit I'm getting from the other substances."*

So garlic is a negative food as it costs our body more to process it that it benefits from it. Now if it tasted sweet and high in glucose, then it would be more benefits in it for us. Lettuce for example has some toxins in it, but there are far more benefits than bad stuff, so it doesn't taste bitter to us and it is valuable as a daily source of vitamins, minerals and alkaline.

Now, when by our own activity and habits we disable our own defense, our bodies get sick and toxic and run down. Our taste buds get sluggish and can't always tell us what we're supposed to be eating, as we'll find out later.

Now let's see what's the difference between real food, for example a carrot and a junk food—*Twinkie,* all American snack cake.

*Real food (carrot) vs. junk food (Twinkie):*

|             | Carrot | Twinkie | Comments |
|-------------|--------|---------|----------|
| Glucose     | yes    | yes     | 1        |
| Protein     | yes    | 1/2     | 2        |
| Fatty acids | yes    | no      | 3        |
| Minerals    | yes    | no      | -        |
| Vitamins    | yes    | no      | 4        |
| Water       | yes    | 1/32    | -        |
| Toxins      | no     | yes     | -        |

*Comments:*

*(1)   Twinkie has glucose as well, sugar is sugar.*

*(2)   Carrot has what's called a "complete protein", Twinkie might have some.*

*(3)   We can analyze that Twinkie and find something that chemically looks like cholesterol or fatty acid (oil), but it's denatured! Once we heat the oil above 44°C (112°F) the chemical structure is altered to what our liver cannot process it and it's not usable by the body. This is the cholesterol that sticks inside the artery wall and cause arteriosclerosis (hardening of arteries).*

*(4)   Whole-wheat bread has around 40 nutrients in it. When flour industry gets to process it, the white refined flour has 0-2 nutrients.*

There's the difference between the real food and the junk food. Junk food is missing part of the package, it's not all there. In order for the body to use the junk food it's going to have to make up the difference.

## How the body makes the difference?

Let's say you've just been out and had your favorite Mexican meal and your body begun to digest. The glucose is extracted from that meal and sent along by the liver into the cells of the body. Then glucose is processed[5] in order to become a usable energy. But the catalyst (vitamins + minerals) must be present in order to convert the glucose. If we eat real food (unprocessed, raw or steamed) it comes as a part of the package.

What happens if we eat junk food deprived of vitamins? How do you get energy form the Twinkie? The answer is that your body will process it drawing what's needed from its reserves. But we were given reserves for emergency situations only.

Imagine, if a mother sees her kid falling into the swimming pool, what would happen immediately? She gets stressed out and her blood pressure spikes up in no time. What's happening? As the adrenaline flows it tells the liver to get some sugar from the cells, necessary to speed up the metabolism, to give mother some energy right now so she can save her little one. Mother didn't have time to go and eat a banana! Those catalysts to process the sugar from cells to give the energy to act had to be present and ready to go. You see now, the emergency system is there for a reason—a short-term emergency support.

For a short time the adrenaline is flowing keeping you alive but it can't go indefinitely, you would die, you don't have enough reserves of catalyst nutrients to keep you going. But the way most people live now is, they run on emergency all the time, and it begins to burn these reserves out.

Now innate intelligence says:

> *"This fellow still wants me to keep him alive but he's not giving me any ingredients, how am I going do it?"*

So it looks at the bones and says:

> *"My, what a wonderful supply of catalysts!"*

and starts to pull out the minerals from those bones—calcium, phosphorus and others, to process the glucose or the protein, through the various cycles.

---

[5] If you want to know more search for information on the *citric acid cycle* outside this book.

Innate intelligence <u>draws from its own tissues to keep the body alive</u>! It strives to keep the body alive regardless of the costs, and the cost is—disease!

# Chapter 3: Toxins and stimulants

Toxin is a substance that our body is not designed to run on. For a while our body can get away with running on fuel that wasn't designed for it but at a cost. Our body begins to slow down as it begins to get diseased.

We have come to believe, because it is so common, that aging is normal. We believe that it is just normal for the person in their 50's-60's having a heart attack or arthritis and things like that. It's not normal, although it's very common.

But the body is not designed to run that way. There are cultures in this world still alive and well documented, living to be a 140-150 years of age in good health, working until just until a few days before death. And all those poor people don't have all those wonderful, refined foods we do! Isn't that too bad? You see, they are living on the right fuel, we are not. And so our bodies begin to pay a price.

Know that garlic won't kill you today, know that a cup of coffee won't kill you today, if it did, nobody would be eating or drinking them. But it's in the long term we are missing the big picture. It will kill you in a long run, it will make you sick.

All toxins are stimulants. What is a **stimulant**? It's anything that revs up the metabolism. Why is the body raving up when we put it this toxin? Because it's trying to get it out of the system, always trying to "clean house".

The most famous and often used stimulant everyone knows is *caffeine*. But did you know that there's enough caffeine in 1 cup of coffee, about 120 mg, to kill you if injected directly to the bloodstream? Why it does not kill you? And where do you get the energy from when you drink a cup of coffee? Don't say *"caffeine"* because we know already that our only source of energy is glucose.

The answer is this. When that coffee hits the stomach the body senses **it's about to be poisoned**, and it sends a signal to adrenal glands and says:

*"Adrenals, tell the liver to get some sugar out!"*

The cells need to take that sugar and convert it to energy to rev up the metabolism to process that caffeine out of the bloodstream right now, before it accumulates and kills us. So adrenaline starts to flow and the glucose level into the bloodstream goes up and the cells get the glucose and they speed up and they save our life, one more time. And during that whole process we feel fantastic, but at what cost? The body had to draw from its reserves to bring up glucose and catalysts, getting all worked up. So soon we'll add another cup of coffee because we feel so tired, and the whole crazy cycle starts again. And next year, because we feel sicker, we will have to add another cup of coffee, instead of one, we drink two or three in the morning.

# How do we compensate the lack of energy?

If the cell is healthy then when we sleep at night it produces a 100% of energy for tomorrow's activities. But let's say this cell is running on 50% of its capacity because of years of abuse through diet, so when you go to bed tonight it manufactures 50% of energy. How do we get thought the day if we only had 50% of energy? Through stimulation the body revs up that 50% to act like a 100% and we run on adrenaline for the rest of the day. And what's the cost of running on adrenaline? Depleting our health even more. So next year we are running at 40% and we have to add more stimulation to make up the difference. And we keep doing that until one day our body can't cover for us anymore and that's when we end up in the doctor's office, saying:

*"Last month I just fell apart."*

You were falling apart for years but adrenaline just wouldn't cover for you anymore.

*Adrenaline revs **up** the metabolism, covering up*
*for the missing energy in the body cells*

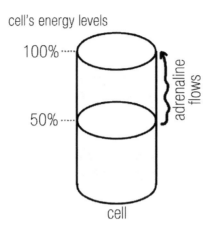

Here is a story that shows what's happening around the world right now. Some scientists took some rats and put them in the fridge. They gave them some water and food and closed the door. The next day they open the door to see the mice were all held together in the corner. They hadn't had any food or water. The next day they opened the fridge—same story, the mice were still held in the corner. When they opened it, on the third day, the mice were running around, eating, acting like everything was normal. Then the scientists said:

*"This is fantastic! They've learned to adapt in this adverse environment!"*

But the next day, when they opened the fridge, all mice were dead. When they opened them up to look inside, they found out that their stress glands and adrenals were completely wasted. What did happen to them?

While trying to adapt to the environment, they were getting revved up, and they compensated and they carried on what may appear as a normal life in the end, but in reality they all got burned out. That's what we see in America and all around the world. People eating fast food, junk food three times a day seem to be in a perfect health until the age 35-40. Then suddenly everything begins to fall apart.

## After a big meal

Now how about feeling sleepy after a big meal? Everyone does, right? Let's find out why. When you eat big meal your sick, exhausted body doesn't have the energy to process and digest all that food, as it takes a lot of energy to do that. The body then "says":

> *"I'm going to have to knock you out to free up this energy that's keeping you conscious, so I can digest the food."*

But what have we learned to do? What's the great American after-dinner habit? Coffee, or a cigarette or dessert or all three, to get those adrenals going so we can stay awake and process and digest our food. We do not give our bodies a break.

One of the best tests you can do to find out how healthy you are is to eat only fruits and vegetables just for one day, drop everything else, and see how far you get. See if you can even get out of bed without that first cup of coffee. If you can't, you know how much adrenaline you are running on.

The great illusion of stimulation is that while we are raved up we think we feel good, and in the mean time we get sicker and sicker.

## How do we know when to stop eating?

When do we know we have enough to eat? It hurts! At least this is the current trend. After a big meal we may feel uncomfortable because our stomach can handle only so much food at the time. Anything above that digestive capacity begins to break down to a rotting process (putrefaction, fermentation) which turns in to toxins, highly poisonous. They don't just pass through unfortunately, but they are absorbed.

So innate intelligence, always trying to keep the body as healthy as possible, may bring this whole meal up, or else, next best would be diarrhea first thing in the morning. That's the body getting toxins out before they are absorbed.

Now that's a symptom—diarrhea. The body's trying to get rid of the toxins. The last thing you want to do is to take a pill to keep those toxins in!

> The symptoms are our friends. That's the body's effort to undo what we did wrong to it.

But where's the energy coming from for that diarrhea? As in everything, it also uses up energy, it's not free. Once again it comes from our reserves, from our body.

# Chapter 4: Inorganic vs. organic

If you get cow's milk, pasteurize it and feed it to its offspring, in 6 months that calf would be dead. Why? That milk had no nutrients any more. The only thing that calf was living on was the glucose in the milk and its own nutrition reserves. As soon as it had burned it all up, it died.

If we were to take an x-ray of a person who had been diagnosed with osteoporosis[6] 10 years before, and if we'd asked him, what he'd been doing about it, he may say that he's been drinking a lot of milk and taking calcium tablets. What's interesting, if you look at the x-ray, you'll discover not only more of the mineral content loss, but you would see calcium deposits outside the bones. Why is the body not taking it inside?

***Calcium deposits*** *outside the bones*

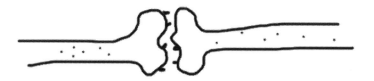

The answer to both of those questions is this:

> The calcium in pasteurized milk is **inorganic**. Our bodies were designed to run on organic or **living nutrients**, not dead nutrients.

---

[6] it's a loss of minerals from the bone

The plant kingdom has the ability to take inorganic nutrients such as calcium, iron, potassium, phosphorus and sodium from the earth and it will add a protein enzyme to them a protein enzyme, making that all one molecule. That's a living, or **organic** nutrient and only the plant kingdom has this ability to provide them.

Remember this, when we eat inorganic substances, our body can't recognize them and use them. If we drink milk and eat dead calcium tablets to fight osteoporosis, remember those are inorganic. We need a catalyst attached, a mineral or a "passport" if you will, to get it into the body to help the body use it. This is true for all the supplements you take.

# Vitamins and supplements— organic vs. synthetic

If you think that by taking supplements you have all necessary nutrition intake covered, better think again. Most of the synthetic substances available in stores, while they work in tests tubes (in vitro) they have no measurable or significant effect on humans. More so, in most cases synthetic products mess up with other nutrient's absorption. Beta-carotene for example, when used in its synthetic form, affects the ability of Vitamin E to work in the body.

Why does a synthetic version of a vitamin not work? Let's take the Vitamin C for example. What typically is called ascorbic acid or Vitamin C in most supplements starts off as corn, becomes corn sugar, then it's processed and isolated and becomes crystal in structure. In its natural form, in a lemon for example, Vitamin C is not crystal in structure at all, but it has a more rounded shape. What does it mean? Those vitamins don't look the same and they don't work the same. They won't be recognized by the body and they won't be used. In the best case they will be expelled from the body, but it's quite common, especially in a toxic and ineffective environment, that they are stored in the body cells.

Remember, the more we process the food the less value is in it.

32

# The hierarchy of food processing

Just to give you an idea about how many nutrients there are in food we eat, I give you the following hierarchy. At this point you should be able to link the level of nutrients content in food with the level of your health.

1. The whole, raw food—that is the most organic food, it has the most life in it. That's how we should eat our food ideally.
2. Juiced and drinking it as soon as it's juiced[7].
3. Dehydrated or dried, without additives—it loses 2-5% of its nutrients value.
4. Freshly picked and frozen immediately—loses between 5-30% of its nutrients value.
5. Steamed[8]—loses 15-60%.
6. Leftovers (raw foods, e.g. a salad prepared the night before, stored in the fridge, even sealed in a container). Once we tear the lettuce it begins oxidizing and loosing nutrients.
7. Cooked, baked, steamed too long —depends on the process and time it loses 40-100%.
8. Cooked leftovers.
9. Microwaved[9]—loses 90-99% of its nutrition value.
10. Commercially canned foods.
11. Fried foods.
12. Foods with additives.

With the last three not only do we lose all nutritional valuable but we start adding toxins. The more money and more intelligence that are put into processing the food, the less value is left in to the body.

---

[7] Once the skin of fruits and vegetables is broken, oxygen combines with the enzymes and kills them, so because of oxidation the juice becomes inorganic. Drink the juice within 30 minutes and a couple of hours to get the most benefit from it.

[8] Steamed means the green is still crispy, if it's limp, it's cooked.

[9] The microwave cooks by bombarding the molecules in the food, causing them to shake around. They start bombarding each other that creates friction, which creates heat, which cooks it. Just this bombardment process, with the molecules hitting each other, breaks off the enzymes attached to the minerals and it becomes inorganic.

# Chapter 5: Disease and healing process

## About pH

Before we can go any further we need to learn about pH. pH is a measurement of how acid or alkaline a substance is and ranges from 0 to 14. pH of 1 is acid, pH of 14 alkaline and pH of 7 is neutral (for example, pure water has a pH of about 7).

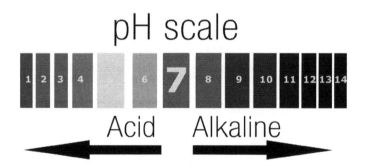

Our bodies work the most efficiently at the range of **pH 7-8** (cell's pH).

As long as we stay within this range we are in good health.

The blood pH is 7.4. If the blood drops e.g. to 7.2 we die!

Since our daily metabolism is acid producing, and our body **can't make an alkaline** material, then we have to find an outside source for it, so we can use it daily to maintain life. Nature provided the way. How do we bring the alkaline into the body? By eating fresh fruits and vegetables.

And you may ask:

*"How about citrus fruits, like oranges, aren't they acid?"*

The answer is that the *citric acid* you find in citrus fruit is an organic acid and that means your body has the ability to take that organic acid and completely metabolize it. If you get that orange and burn it in the lab, you'd get an ash that would be alkaline. However, if we do the same with meat, the ash that would be leftover would be acid. Meat has some inorganic acid (phosphoric and sulfuric acid), that we cannot process.

# How do we get sick?

The body's normal metabolism is acid producing and so we should be replenishing the alkaline every day. Just to give you a perspective. In order for the body just to neutralize the inorganic acid of one steak, it's going to take 9 meals; 3 days of eating just raw fruits and vegetables. How are we going to keep the body alkaline if our normal daily metabolism is going acid, plus we are eating primarily acid diet?

Let's first look at the average acid-forming foods in the body, listed from the least to the most acidic.

*The acid-forming foods:*

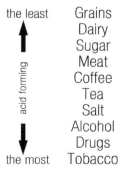

35

How does the blood stays at the pH of 7.4, in spite of all that acid we are putting in? You don't have to be a chemist to understand you cannot continue dumping the acid into the body and stay alkaline, it won't happen. Yet somehow it stays that for a long time. If you would go to the doctor to check your blood pH it's always going to be at 7.4. If your blood drops to just 7.35 for a very long time you start turning blue, and they will put you in an oxygen tent.

What does the standard American diet (SAD) look like and how much of that is alkaline?[10]

---

### *Standard American Diet (SAD)*

#### *Breakfast:*
- *bacon and eggs, toast, orange juice (out of the can), coffee*

#### *Mid-morning:*
- *coffee, a donut*

#### *Lunch:*
- *hamburger and fries, coke (let's not forget about the lettuce and tomato in that burger—it's being laying all day and oxidizing)*

#### *Mid-afternoon:*
- *coke and a candy bar*

#### *Dinner:*
- *meat and potatoes, maybe some canned vegetables*
- *dessert: ice cream, a pie or a cake*

---

Do you know the average American goes 7-14 days without having any fruits and vegetables what so ever? How in the world does the body stay alive? To keep the blood in the pH of 7.4, the alkaline is being pulled out from the cell, from its own tissue.

---

[10] Alkaline are fresh and raw fruit and vegetables.

*The cell will give up the alkaline material*
*to keep the blood at pH of 7.4*

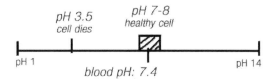

The cell can get away with the pH less than 7-8, but it's not in good health any more, and the cell is not functioning as efficiently as it was designed to. It can get as low as a pH of 3.5 and then it's so inefficient it quits, and we call it death.

*The cell will give up the alkaline material*
*until its gets to as low as pH of 3.5, when it gives up and dies*

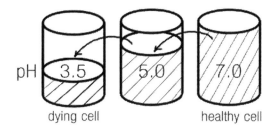

Disease starts anywhere below pH of 7, although we wouldn't name it disease at that point yet. We would just slow down and we'd be a little sluggish. It's a common aging process we've talked about earlier but it's not normal to age, instead—it's normal to grow older.

Cancer **can't exist** in the cell pH of **5.8** or higher

Research shows that the pH of the average American cell is between pH of 5-5.5. It's no wonder we are on an express train to chronic, degenerative disease: cancer, arthritis, diabetes, heart disease. 80% of Americans over the age of 40 have a chronic degenerative disease. That's changed rapidly after the 1900's. The more acid the cell is, the less efficiently it does what it was supposed to do. If it is a heart cell it doesn't

37

"heart" so well, and so we call it a disease. The taste buds are not immune, they are also becoming acid and they can no longer tell us what foods are good and which ones aren't. The acid food starts to taste good. I give you an example.

Do you remember the first time you had a coffee? I bet you had to have some sugar to get it down, because your taste buds were telling you not to put that in, it's bad for you! But as we get sicker and our bodies more sluggish the body need that stimulation, if we want to feel as good as we did the last year. So we start drinking more and more coffee and the body's pH keeps dropping lower and lower.

## What's the answer to health?

Why we don't feel good even if our blood looks good? You go to the doctor to check your blood, the results come in and all looks normal? Why do we feel sick?

Because our cells not only will give up alkaline but they will give up other nutrients trying to keep that blood as healthy as possible, because if blood get too sick we die. The cells can get away in lessen health, our blood can't. So what is the answer to health? How do we return that body to its pH of 7-8? It's very simple—by adding alkaline back to the body, by adding raw fruits and vegetables to our diet!

I do not recommend you to stop eating all the acid-forming foods at once, since you depend on them. It is very important how you start and I will guide you through that process step by step (read more: *Further readings: It's important how you start*).

# The disease process

Now when we understand what alkaline is, we can talk about the actual disease process and how important this material is to keep us in good health. How is it that we are developing colds, flu or cancer? Let's start with the symptom.

# What's a symptom?

If we looked up at the ceiling and saw a watermark, we'd decide to fix it. So we get some paint, and we paint—that watermark and it's "fixed". Next time it rains what happens? The watermark is back. So we decide to take some serious precautions and seal it. As an analogy to that it would be like taking a stronger drug for your headache, if the aspirin didn't help.

Now, the next time it rains that original stain didn't return, but we have a mark all around the sealed area. That's a whole new disease, isn't it? We cured the first one. To continue with our analogy—it's now the time for surgery. So we get the saw, we cut out that whole part of the ceiling and we replace it. And it'll work for a while, but as the rain continues falling the watermark is back on the ceiling. None of us would be so ignorant when it comes to the leaking roof. We would go up to the roof and we'd fix it in the first place, right? But when it comes to our health we are that ignorant unfortunately.

We think the symptom is the enemy. In fact the symptom is our friend trying to keep us alive, and overcome the wrong that we did. Remember when I mentioned diarrhea? That was a symptom and our body's attempt to remove the toxins that we ate.

# How do we handle toxins?

After our taste buds get sluggish and they do not recognize toxic food for us anymore, it's up to the liver to keep those toxins out of the body. The liver will initially try to neutralize those toxins with alkaline. The poison come in but it just neutralizes it with alkaline and sends them out through the blood, kidneys, lungs, back to the liver, out through the bowel.

*Liver gives up its own alkaline material to neutralize toxin*
*and sends it away*

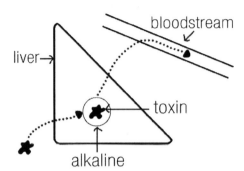

But it doesn't take the liver long to realize that in order to survive it can't give up all its reserves. So it comes up with another solution. The liver hangs on to them, which doesn't cost it any alkaline, but the price is that it becomes more toxic or congested and less efficient, and we begin to slow down a bit.

*Liver stores toxins until it reaches up to 70% of its congestion*

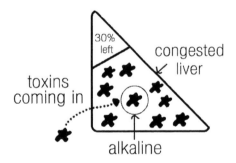

When it reaches the point when the liver gets about 70% congested and it can no longer hang to those toxins at this rate. If it could, it would fill up and die. So it starts giving those toxins out to the bloodstream, and as soon as it does, the body's cells react in less than a second, giving away their own alkaline.

*Congested liver cannot store any more toxins—it sends it to bloodstream*
*where toxins are being neutralized by alkaline coming from the cells*

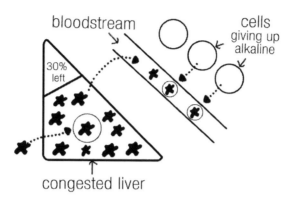

But very soon cells realize what liver had figured out and they "make a deal" with the bloodstream. Instead of getting rid of the alkaline in such a quick paste, they start storing those toxins inside and all around them. That way, toxins are out of the blood stream which can now safely maintain its pH of 7.4. But at what price?

*A state of toxicity—toxins are stored in and around cells in the body*

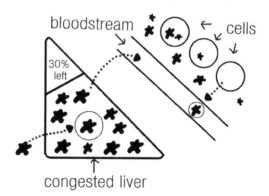

That is called **a state of toxicity** and is defined as a part of the body that stores toxins that it wasn't designed to do so. There's no place in the body that is designed to store toxins. There are only two places designed to store a waste products and only temporarily and that is the bowel and the bladder. In a state of toxicity the cells are going to react against these toxins being there. That reaction is called disease or illness—the cells will fight back as they were not designed to store any of that material in there.

# How do we get a summer cold?

Starting around the end of October we begin to eat a lot more junk food during Halloween, Thanksgiving and Christmas. Parties, big dinners, less sunshine, less fruits and vegetables, cold air (another stress to the body), and you start slowing down, while the level of toxication of our bodies is starting to go higher and higher. Imagine your sinus membrane filling up with toxins your body doesn't know what to do with, until it gets full enough that your body will try to get it out. Then we have something called "a cold." No one ever catches a cold, you earn it.

So why is it, when you get a cold, there are people who eat and live in worst conditions that you do, who do not get a cold? Why is it that people with cancer don't get a cold in often two or three years? It doesn't make sense, right? A lack of cold is considered to be healthy. No, it takes energy to have a cold! You do not feel very energetic while having a cold though because your body's focusing on the cleansing process, trying to push these toxins out.

*When in early November I switched to a raw food diet and I started exercising, in spring already I had my first flu. I couldn't understand why now? After all my body's chemistry was improving and it was spring after all! Addicted to an early coffee and greasy junk food before the transition, my body couldn't afford the energy to get sick, it was too busy dealing with the daily input of variety of toxins. When I changed my lifestyle and my body got more rest and more nutrients in, it was ready to do it. That's where the summer cold came from. So if you don't have a winter cold, you better hope you have a summer cold.*

If you are healthy enough you won't have these toxins in there, so you won't have any colds, but it's the very, very sick people who don't get those colds, because the body is too sick and weak to push it out. As it loses vitality it can no longer afford the house cleansing.

# What is an infection?

Louis Pasteur said to us that germs cause a disease. Now he had a contemporary by the name of Van Camp, who said, "You're right, germs do cause disease, but not in the way you are telling us." Pasteur was telling us that as we walk the road these bacteria just

42

attack us and we catch a disease. Van Camp said, "No, we have to give that bug a reason to be there, germs are scavengers, they live on toxins, not healthy tissue. We first have to make the body sick by what we are eating, before the germs have any effect." On his death bed, Louis Pasteur admitted that Van Camp was right.

You can catch a bug and if your environment is toxic, you can develop an infection, but just like with a cold, you need to have enough energy first. Before your body will allow for this bug to take over and start producing infection, it must know if it has enough energy. First, if it has enough nutrients to get through that time, and that could be from three to seven days of running an infection. And during that time your body is going to want to fast. It's also going to run a fever.

# What is a fever?

The virus in our body is producing a poison which is toxic to the body, and our body will have to rev up our metabolism drastically to get that poison out of our body before it kills us. That is the fever—the increased metabolism. Who produced the fever? The body, trying to keep up with the bacteria. What was the germ doing there? Just doing some "house cleaning" feasting on toxins we've stored. So if you are healthy enough to run an infection you can expect a fever. This is your body's way of dealing with the bacteria inside. If the temperature is too high you can try to bring it down with a sponge bath or a cool enema, but not with drugs.

Now, I don't know how about you, but it seems to me that if the body wanted the fever up there, let's keep it there. People die of infections when we try to bring the temperature down. Now the bacteria have the best time, there's nothing to keep them in check!

# How does an antibiotic work?

Doctors know if you use antibiotics for a long time, they need to start monitoring the liver functions, because the liver will start to shut down. What an antibiotic does is it draws energy from the infection to the liver so the body has to make a decision, either it's going to keep the liver alive or it will continue the infection process, there's no enough energy to do both. The liver is more important so the body separates that germ, puts it into "a pocket" to keep it on hold until the time is right to get back to the cleansing process, and then moves the energy to the liver to deal with that antibiotic. What we observe is the symptom going away, but the germ is still there, sometimes for years, waiting to be dealt with.

*Body isolates the germ, putting the infection on hold*

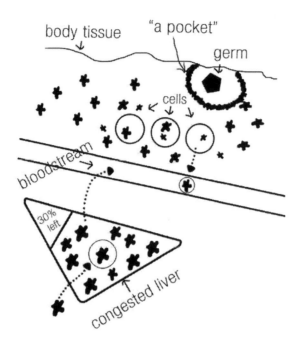

# How to get through the sickness?

With calm mind, resting and fasting ideally. Your body wants to fast and rest during the process of cleansing. It will focus all the energy, revving your metabolism to generate a high fever and all you need to do is let it do what it does the best and rest. I know it can be scary in the beginning, to have a little faith and stay away from drugs, but please try at least one day if you can, and you'll be better off already. The next time when the fever comes back, try two days of fasting and resting, as your faith improves. Let the body do what it does best without interfering with the process.

# Is cancer inevitable?

If you say, "but I have to get back to work so I need those drugs to put me on my feet" that's fine, it's your decision. But be aware what you are doing to yourself. Not only are you putting on hold the cleansing process and letting them stay in your body, but you are also adding new toxins. And so you can take the drug and continue getting more toxic and more sluggish by eating what you've been eating, getting more acid and sick, losing vitality. The day will come when those cells will no longer be able to push toxins out through the body and they begin to just hold the toxins there. That's when it begins to develop what is called a *chronic degenerative disease*. The tissues now begin to scar, to deform and they begin to mutate, which is called a cancer. That's what a cancer is— the end disease of all diseases.

Cancer is the end disease of all diseases.

## How does it begin?

If we would look at a cell in the body that's going to make a new cell, the cell is going to divide in the middle and the genes will split apart and two new cells emerge.

*Cell's dividing*

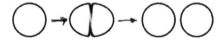

Are those cells healthy if the mother cell was toxic? Of course not, all they did was split down the middle. Let's say it's a lung area and this person smokes cigarettes, and so his body will be acid but the lung tissues will be extremely acid because of the direct input of the nicotine in there. As this cell begins to divide, those genes get confused and what is born are deformed or "crazy" cells because the genetic code was messed up.

*Toxic cell is dividing*

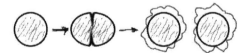

That's how we create cancer cells. They all have the same characteristics, regardless of where they are found in the body—they do not know what they are, they act on their own. They just keep eating, growing and multiplying. They don't know any more whether they are heart cells or liver cells or lung cells.

I'll say it again—**cancer is the end disease of all diseases**, and if we stay alive long enough eating a toxic diet, we'll all get cancer. Right now things like heart attack or diabetes is killing us first but that's changing quickly.

# Development of a chronic disease

What was the reason for storing the toxins in and around cells again? To keep them away from the bloodstream, to keep us alive. The long-term result of that was development of a disease. But what is a chronic disease? We live from one disease to another, thinking that we are keeping ourselves healthy by taking medications, whilst we are developing a chronic condition. How?

*The development of the chronic disease*

cold  we take a drug for that,
      not allowing the body to cleanse
as we continue to get toxic we develop something called

bronchitis  and we start taking drug for that
*that's adifferent disease we think now but it's the same, just more severe*
and after medicating brinchitis we develop

asthma

again we take another medication,
we continue eating the same toxic food
and we develop what we call

congestive heart failure

# How does the drug work?

How do they take away the symptoms and makes us feel better? If you ask a pharmacist how aspirin works he would tell you it has a numbing effect on the entire being, because if you have a headache or toe ache, it makes the symptom go away, except if you have a stomach pain. It doesn't make sense, does it? If it has a numbing effect on the entire body, surely it'd take care of the stomach. After all it's a part of the body, right? That's one of the mysteries of the aspirin.

Let's say you were out in the garden and you got a thorn in your finger, so you decided to go back home, take the tweezers and get it out but on your way back you step on the nail. Would you remember the thorn in your finger? No! Is it healed? Of course not, but you got distracted as your body shifted its attention from the finger to the foot—something more important going on there, something more life threatening.

Well every aspirin causes a teaspoon of bleeding in the stomach, if it didn't cause the bleeding it wouldn't work.

## What causes a headache?

Generally a headache is caused from the blood being too toxic. So when we take an aspirin that causes bleeding in the stomach, which do you think is more life threatening—toxic blood or internal bleeding? Internal bleeding, you are right. So the body shifts its attention from head to stomach. Now if that aspirin did not take care of the pain then you take six aspirin—now you have more life-threatening situation for sure.

All drugs work in a similar manner—they create a disease of their own.

Drugs are always shifting attention from the symptoms you've been complaining to your doctor about. But your body will try to throw them off and sometimes we experience symptoms of them, we call side effects. Skin breaks out in a rush—the body's dumping toxins out through the skin. You get kind of drowsy—it's the same process when you are going under anesthesia; that gas is so toxic to the body, it can't keep you both awake and alive, it has to knock you out to process the gas that's going to kill you otherwise.

# The logic behind taking drugs

If you could take any drug you like and give it to a healthy person, they'll become sick. What is that sickness? It's the body trying to throw off that poison. But here is what we are doing—we are giving the same drug, the poison to a sick person and we expect them to get healthy. Is that logical to you? Now, I'm not telling you to stop taking your drugs tomorrow, your body may be depend on those for life! Rather that, as you improve your diet and your body's chemistry as your body returns to health, you'll find your body doesn't need them. That's the decision that you have to make.

# The processed-foods era

## The Pottenger experiment

Back in the 40s a dentist by the name of Francis Pottenger wanted to find out what processed foods do to the body. What's important to know is that Francis Pottenger financed his own research. You may also want to know that he wasn't a good example of perfect health. Pottenger took about 800 cats and he divided them into five groups. The first two he fed with natural, wholesome food, while the other three groups he fed with a processed junk food and he started to observe.

In the first two groups every generation lived in good health. One day they got worned out, and they died, as they were supposed to. But with the junk-food-fed cats that wasn't the case. By the end of the first generation, the junk-food cats began to develop diseases, cancer, arthritis, flues, allergies, colds. The second generation of junk-food cats began to develop the same diseases in the middle of their lifetime. The third generation junk-food cats began to develop those diseases at birth or shortly after. Many of them were born deformed and very lethargic. If you held them and dropped they wouldn't turn over, they just fell, they had no fight, no spunk. The calcium content of their bones was next to nothing. There was no fourth generation! Either the third generation was sterile or they aborted their offspring.

## Conclusion

Right now in America 35% of young adults is sterile. There are more spontaneous abortions, miscarriages than there ever was before. Do you know what the number one leading cause of death of children under the age of 10 in America is? Cancer. How can that be? Those kids haven't been around long enough to get as toxic as their grandparents were (to get cancer). They don't have to be. In each generation that genetic code is getting a little bit weaker and weaker, and it takes less to let those diseases come to the surface. Children develop heart diseases by the age of 15, diagnosed at birth with diabetes, hypoglycemic. These are diseases that were unheard of in 1900's, in children. They are predicting that at the next generation cancer will be epidemic. That's depressing, but it doesn't have to be.

Let me show you some statistics presenting how our diet has changed since the 1900.

- Fresh fruit and vegetables: decreased from 40% to 20%
- Beef consumption: increased 75%
- Cheese consumption: increased 400%
- Fat and oil consumption: increased 150%
- Margarine consumption: increased 800%
- Corn syrup consumption: increased 400%
- Sugar consumption: increased 50%
- Processed fruit and vegetables consumption: increased 400%

*(data showing consumption changes between 1900 and 1980)*

Now if you combine these statistics with a weakening genetic code, you can see why America is in an epidemic of chronic degenerative diseases.

# What determines who gets what disease?

## a. Inherent genetic weakness

We do not inherit a disease, we inherit a potential. If we live a life our parents do, we too will develop the same condition. It's up to us and our choices.

## b. Health of the parents

When the child was conceived. Parents, I advise if you plan a child, do 3-months clean up before, to give the little one a good start.

## c. Health of the mother while carrying child

If the mother is not healthy she will compete with the babe for nutrients and energy (the child can get aborted).

## d. What a mother eats is important

What she eats makes a babe, so if she eats junk, she's going to grow a "junk babe."

### e. What a mother eats while nursing a babe

What she eats affects the milk the babe is fed with. Any toxins she eats will be shared with the babe often affecting the babe with diarrhea, vomiting or colic.

# The healing crisis

Let's talk about healing. What happens when you begin to put the alkaline foods into your system? What does the body do with that? How does that return us to health? What is the mechanism that takes place in cleansing and what can you expect?

Let's look one more time at the situation inside the body. The liver is congested with toxins up to 70% and the cells have toxins in and around them. Now we begin to put the alkaline to the body and the body sends it out to the cells. The cells use it to neutralize toxins and they say to the liver:

*"Here you go, you can pass it through the bloodstream now, it's safe."*

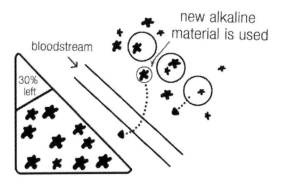

But the liver responds:

*"Thank you cells, I see what you are trying to do up there, I appreciate it but I'm just barely keeping this body alive as it is. If I take this additional task on, I will shut down."*

*That's the reason people die when they fast after just 5 to 10 days, sometimes less. It's because the body dumps so much toxin on the liver during that fast, this toxic liver can't process and it shuts down. You shouldn't go for a prolonged fast without preparing your body and being supervised.*

So what's happening instead? The liver says to cells:

> *"Remember the sinus membrane? Why don't we start dumping those toxins out there?"*

And as a result we have what we call a healing crisis or a cleansing cold. What's the difference between this cold and the one you were having over the Christmas? That was a survival cold. That is as if you had a glass and you are filling it up and it just over flowed. What we are doing now is we are emptying the glass. We've stopped putting in the poisons but the body still has to clean out the mucus membrane. That is a cleansing cold. It's still a cold but it may feel a little different. Some say they feel like they are in control.

There are other things that appear during the healing crisis—the symptoms of the body dumping toxins in a big way such as diarrhea, that's the liver opening up or chest cold, kicking the mucus out of the lungs. It may be something different but wait till it happens and you will know it's a crisis. The body, for the first few weeks is going to gear up, getting the energy ready to go, and finally when it has enough, it goes to it and cleans it out.

# Get ready for reactivation

There's another process of healing called *reactivation*. If you've been covering up your symptoms with medications your whole life, putting the healing on hold, you didn't really expect your body to forget about all that, did you? When your body will have enough energy and will be strong enough, it will get you 5, 10, 20 years back, to those old injuries and infections, to clean the house once and for all. Trust your body and let it work its way, for you just need to rest and fast during the healing process through the history of your sometimes life-time diseases.

This means you will get sick again and if you had a heart attack you may have another, but this time a healing one. If you had an infection treated with antibiotics, even if when you were a child, you may get it back now, as your body will try to get those intruders out. Your ankle was injured and not healed properly? It may start to hurt again during your body's attempt to fix it when the time is right.

Again, the body will not go through it until it has the energy to do it and it doesn't feel safe. Also know that the body heals in cycles of 3 and 7 days, sometimes multiples of that—of 10, maybe 14, 21 days, but that's rare. Be brave and allow your body to do what it was designed to do. Your job is just to create perfect conditions for healing so when the crisis hits you your job is done for now. Just relax and be aware, the body's cleansing and give it all the time it needs. The worst thing you can do is to take another drug to suppress it.

## Internal healing crisis

Do you have to go through everything you ever had? I don't know, it's up to the body. I will tell you, the body does something called internal healing. The crisis hits as you are going along doing pretty good on your diet, than you have a week when you are just dragging. No real symptoms anywhere, you are just tired—that's the internal healing crisis, the body is cleansing something from the inside. You don't always know what your body's working on, but again, you won't go through it until you are both emotionally and physically ready to handle it.

### Easing the pain during the healing crisis

To the degree you ease the pain, to that degree you will slow down the healing. Weigh up your priorities and do what you feel is right for you, just be aware what it means and what's happening.

# Incurable diseases

I believe that every disease is curable with the right approach and diet, but not everybody is curable. Some diseases have such a momentum going, that if we start with the diet, it doesn't get into it before the disease kills the body. If we could keep that body alive long enough, it could cure the disease. What heals the body then, is it the diet? No, it's the body's ability to take this diet and put it to work. But if there's a really sick, diseased body, with the momentum going there's not enough time for the diet to work. But to me it's always worth to try. What's the alternative?

What the medical profession often calls incurable disease is only because they have yet to learn to get out of the body's way and give it a chance to heal itself. They keep trying to drug it into health. How can you poison something into health? Health does not come in a bottle, it comes from within.

# Weight loss game

In the beginning of this book I told you I will tell you why calories have very little to do with getting fat. What does the world calorie mean? Energy. We have two types of calories—acid and alkaline ones. The acid calorie is a toxic calorie. Now, if the body doesn't need that calorie, which it never does, and that calorie is an excess, the body will take that calorie with its toxin and store it as a fat molecule. Other people will store it in the heart, as a heart disease, and so on. This depends on genetic makeup—different people store toxins in different ways. Skinny doesn't necessary mean healthy. If it's an alkaline energy the body will use that energy for cleansing.

Here's a fellow, on a 1000-calorie diet a day and he's gaining weight. When he started consuming 5000 alkaline calories, coming from raw fruits and vegetables, he started losing weight. How can you eat so many calories from just fruits and vegetables—by juicing it into approximately four liters (a gallon) of juice. Thanks to the alkaline healing calories, the body's using the energy to get rid of the toxins. Weight loss is a side benefit of getting healthy.

*Read more on related topic—**Eating enough for weight loss** and **Digestion is distracting** chapters, **Further readings** section.*

# How long does it take to get healthy?

How long did it take you to get sick? The change is not going to happen overnight. 10-days cleansing programs are great but they are not cleaning you totally, not even a tenth, they're just getting you started.

Know that if you can jump in with both feet and be on just fruits and vegetables, take off from work, you'll be in the bed most of the time, cause you are missing the stimulation, you can probably get cleaned out in about three years. But you can do it slower and it will take you five or maybe ten years to get completely clean.

Some will say they would rather continue drinking their coffee and eating their meat and pies and be happy. That's their decision. But I'd rather do a little bit better every day than not. I've got to go through the day anyway. And in ten years from now I will be ten years healthier, than I am today. Why spend the last twenty years in a wheelchair? It's not worth it to me.

# Further readings

# It's important how you start

I do not advise to wake up one day and stop eating all the acid foods. In about three days you won't be able to get up from bed, and you will look for coffee again. If your body is used to running on stimulation it is dependent on it, and if you start up tomorrow, you will soon know what your true level of health is.

Instead, start slowly by adding more alkaline—fruits and vegetables to your diet. The emphasis is not on taking away, it's rather on adding to. We all like to eat more, so it should be easy. If you eat 90% acid 10% alkaline, next month add another 10% of alkaline. How? Add a fruit for breakfast, have a salad before your meal (read more in chapter: *Transition diet*), and have that salad every time you eat. Eat the salad first! Why?

# Appetite and satisfaction

What determines appetite and satisfaction while you're eating? Is it not how full we feel, although we got used to determine it this way. If you make a ham sandwich with white bread, you would be able to eat about five or six of them before your stomach gets full and you will start feeling pain. But if you do this with whole-wheat bread, you may notice the same feeling after just two sandwiches. What made the difference?

It was the **nutrient content**, the quality, not the quantity was different in both of those sandwiches. When we are eating junk food our body is trying to register nutrients, and it keeps asking for more, so you would put something worth eating. So you keep eating until your stomach hurts and now you can't eat anymore, you're full. That's why I advise to eat your salad first, eat the quality first (read more in the **Transition diet**).

Soon you will realize that your appetite for the acid foods drops and now you eat only 80%—it's easy. And the next month you add another 10% of alkaline (now its 70/30) and it keeps dropping, it's a gradual process.

> Once we improve the body chemistry, once the cells' pH starts moving towards alkaline, it starts generating necessary energy itself, instead of relying on the stimulation to get through the day.

And soon you will start cutting from the list all the acid-forming foods you were dependent on (see page 38). First, you will notice, the craving for the cigarettes is gone. Then you would probably put aside some of the drugs. Next, you will realize the alcohol burns and you won't feel like drinking it. Everything will start taste very salty, so you will reduce the amount you use or start skipping it. Coffee, instead of putting you to sleep will keep you awake at night. Next, you will notice you can't stand the smell of meat.

> *What gives meat its taste and aroma when it's cooking? It's the toxins in the meat. A field-grazed cow doesn't have the antibiotics injected in it, doesn't have any of that powerful chemical food they feed it, so it grows fast and big to get quick to the market shelves. Those cows don't have much taste in it. It's these toxic cows that have all the taste. Liver for example, is the worst tasting part of the beef! Why? What does the liver do for the body? It's the primary filter to keep toxins out of the system. That liver is full of poisons, don't ever eat liver!*

Soon you become sensitive to the rest of acid foods. You will notice that sugar gives you a headache, dairy products make mucus in your throat the next morning, sinuses start draining, and grains makes you feel heavy and bloated. But I'm not telling you to give up anything. I'm telling you to add more fruits and vegetables.

When you start adding more fruits and vegetables to your diet you can make a deal with yourself, not to give up your most favorite food, like Mexican food for example, to quiet this overwhelming craving for the hot sauce. You don't have to give is up and you can eat enough alkaline to compensate for the acid you ate. In other words, if you are eating 20% acid and 80% alkaline, you can maintain the cell pH at 7-8. It will be enough alkaline coming in to neutralize the acid you are eating plus maintain cell pH.

> If you are eating only 20% acid and <u>80% alkaline</u>, you can maintain the healthy cell pH at 7-8.

Start eating fruit for breakfast, fruit for snacks and salads for meals, aside of whatever else you are going to eat. In few months your cravings for the Mexican food will start going away, as you will go to your favorite restaurant less frequently that you used to and you realize you are going to there out of habit than to satisfy your taste buds. More often you will feel sluggish immediately after the meal that was heavy and brought toxins in. And if you don't want to become a vegetarian, don't worry. Just add more good to your body and listen to its needs. In time you may realize that, even if you didn't make a conscious choice about it, you haven't have meat or cheese in a long time.

# Eating enough for weight loss

I said before that losing weight is an effect of dumping waste which is being stored in you body together with fat. As your body's chemistry starts improving as a side effect of becoming healthy, your body is losing excess fat. For that to happen though it's important to eat enough raw fruits and vegetables—food that is both nutritious and hydrating. It's challenging to eat enough to keep you satisfied, but crucial, if you want to win with junk food cravings and temptations.

As you are trying to eat more fruit and vegetable-based meals throughout the day, you will notice you get hungry much faster. That's because you are used to eating cooked meals which are usually much smaller, water-depleted and calorie-dense, compared to a fruit meal. It will take some time, usually from 30-60 days before you'll feel comfortable with eating large amount of fruit and raw veggie meals, until you establish a new habit.

Plant-based, raw meals, especially vegetable-based, are low in calorie and high in water. For that reason, you will get full really fast, without having the half of your calorie needs in. It will take some time until you learn how much you need to eat to get you through the day. Be patient. Eat more raw fruits and vegetables as snacks and together with your meals, make smoothies and you will get there.

For example on a 2000 kcal diet, you would eat a breakfast of 700 kcal. That would be:
- about 6,5 medium bananas or
- 4 bananas and 3 Medjool dates or
- 3 bananas, 1 apple, 1 pear and 2 Medjool dates (see also the *Green smoothie* recipe, page 63)

Know that vegetables have very little calories and it's best to eat them with a fat-based dressing to get your calories in (see *Dressing recipes*, pages 64-65). Fat-based meals would ideally be prepared for dinner, as they slow you down and it's not that easy to be active after.

In the same time, fruits can be eaten from breakfast until dinner, giving you all the energy you need to keep up with your activities throughout the day. Eat them ripe and fresh for breakfast, lunch and as a snack. Mix them with greens for highly-nutritious smoothies and enjoy the vitality they bring to your life.

There are many guides available in internet that will help your transition to a raw food diet, adding more to your daily meals and eventually lose weight. I recommend sticking to a low-fat diet such as the 80/10/10, that's been proven to work for everyone who's doing it right. Don't forget to check out guides and programs to help you to transition available on the SweetVeganNature.com too! In the beginning you may want to learn a little bit about how much calories each fruit and veggie has, just to make sure you are eating enough. I highly recommend one tool that has it all—visit free website chronometer.com for all data about the nutrition content broken into carbohydrates, protein and fats, vitamins and minerals, into nice charts.

Do not worry about eating more than you need in the transition period, as it's perfectly fine. Your body will be happy that it gets so much quality food, it will store the extra energy for when it's ready to clean the house (remember, we talked about the healing crisis). Then it will burn the saved energy to dump the waste you've been storing around the belly or other. What's important is to eat enough so you are not hungry, for a successfully transition and notice the results.

# Transition diet

## Smoothie for breakfast

If you could improve just one small thing in your diet, I always recommend changing the breakfast. Smoothie for breakfast is, in my opinion the second best after the whole and juicy fruit. They also create a great opportunity to add extra alkaline, such as lettuce or celery that will blend, leaving you with a beautiful green color and a mouthful meal.

### Green smoothie

My favorite is a smoothie made of:
- 3 bananas
- 1 apple and 1 pear
- 2 Medjool dates for extra sweetness
-  and a celery stalk with 4-5 lettuce leaves for super alkaline content

Mix with a bit of water and enjoy! That's about 700 calories and a perfect meal for breakfast. Drink it slowly but try to drink it in one sitting. The longer smoothie oxidizes the less nutrients in it.

### Fruit smoothie

All these smoothies you can mix and match, ideally respecting the guidelines outlined in the food combination section. If you want, add some water or coconut water. I like adding celery to all my smoothies, it's a green miracle for our bodies and great source of alkaline. Try my favorite combinations of fruit smoothies or come up with your own.

- mango and oranges
- strawberries and oranges
- blueberries and apricots
- peaches and papaya
- raspberries and bananas
- plums, dates and cherries

# Salad and dressing recipes

Dressing recipes are super easy to make using your blender or food processor. In the raw food kitchen they are often of the dip consistency, to spread or massage through the salad leaves and chopped veggies.

What to make your salads from? Green or red-leaf lettuce is a great base to start. Use at least half a head for your side dish and a whole one, if for a single meal. Chop a tomato or two, half of cucumber, or zucchini, maybe one more veggie you love and prepare your dressing. Try not mixing too many ingredients—it's going to digest easier and faster. For the creamy and nutritious dressing use one of unprocessed, natural fats such as: avocado, almonds, sesame seeds, coconut oil or flaxseed. Ideally, chose one at the time. Remember about soaking your nuts and seeds accordingly before eating them, to enable its digestion.

## Sour avocado dressing

- handful of lettuce leaves
- handful of cilantro and/or parsley
- juice of 2 lemons or limes
- 1 avocado
- 2 stalks of celery

- handful of cherry tomatoes
- 3-4 sundried tomatoes
     (soaked if very dry)
- ½ cup of green onions (optional)

Blend all in food processor or in a blender, starting on a low-speed mode. Add a bit of water if necessary.

## Sesame dressing

- handful of lettuce leaves
- a cup of sesame seeds
     (soaked overnight)
- juice of 2 lemons
- 1 stalk of celery

- medium cucumber
- handful of dill
- slice of fresh ginger
- 1 Medjool date or few raisins

Blend all in food processor or in a blender, starting on a low-speed mode. Add a bit of water if necessary.

## Tomato dressing / marinara sauce

- 2 large ripe tomatoes
- a cup of cherry tomatoes
- 2 Medjool dates
  or one tablespoon of raisins
- 3-4 sundried tomatoes
  (soaked if very dry)

- 3-4 tablespoons of tamarind sauce
  (optional)
- a cup of fresh basil
- handful of fresh oregano
  (optional)
- 1-2 tablespoons of coconut oil

Blend all in food processor or in a blender, starting on a low-speed mode. For the Marinara sauce you want a thicker consistency, therefore leave it in a strainer to drain of the juices. Drink the juice and use the sauce for your recipe.

# Main dishes

Main dish can be as simple as salad or as complex as lasagne. You will find thousands of recipes all over the internet, so I will share just a few of the easiest and my recent favourites.

## Thai noodles

For the mixed noodles you can use:

- coconut noodles (scooped out from the coconut with fork or a special tool)
- zucchini noodles (make the noodles using a kitchen appliance called *spiralizer* or *spiral slicer*, available in stores online)

For the sauce:

- 1 tomato
- ¼ cup of papaya
- ¼ cup of avocado
- juice of 1 lemon and 1 lime

- 3 tablespoons of tamarind sauce
- slice of ginger, minced (optional)
- 2 tablespoons of coconut water
- pinch of chopped fresh cilantro

Blend sauce ingredients all together and pour over the noodles. Enjoy.

# Veggie wraps with guacamole

To prepare guacamole you need:

- avocado
- lime juice
- tomato

- ½ of small onion or a handful of chopped green onions

Process all ingredients in a food processor.

For veggie wraps chose your favourite veggies, chopped in julienne style (long, thin strips), I like using:

- carrots
- cucumbers
- red bell peppers

- tomatoes
- sprouts

To wrap your veggies with guacamole you need some sort of a green leaf, such as collard or large kale leaf. It can also be a romaine leaf, in which you can eat it *taco style*— unwrapped. Sometimes I like wrapping in a cabbage leaf, white and/or red, it makes my meal extra crispy. Occasionally, even though it's not raw, I would use rice paper. I do not use nori sheets (seaweed) anymore (read about seaweed on page 70), but it's up to you if you want to experiment.

# Veggie burgers

Very often this recipe is dehydrated, bringing the taste to a new level, but it is also very successful, and quick, when eaten fresh.
For the burger patties you will need:

- 2 large carrots, ground
- 1 stalk of celery
- 4-5 sundried tomatoes
  (soaked, if very dry)

- pumpkin seeds
  (ideally, soaked for 4 hours)
- green onions (optional)

Process all ingredients in a food processor until well combined. Next, using hands, form 3-4 balls, depending on the desired burgers size, and by one, press the balls down to form round-shaped patties.

Burgers can be eaten on dehydrated bread, with lettuce, slice tomato and cucumber, some sprouts and with raw ketchup or other sauce. You can also eat it just wrapped in a green leaf such as romaine, collards or kale, or try in a Portobello mushroom.

## Raw ketchup recipe

To make raw ketchup, follow the Tomato/Marinara Sauce you will find among the dressing recipes, but scoop the tomato seeds before blending, to keep it denser. You can add a teaspoon of apple cider vinegar for the ketchup-like taste.

## White sauce recipe

If you want to try other sauce for the burger, blend 1 cup of sunflower seeds (soaked overnight) with ¾ cup of water and some lemon juice. Add a piece of onion and some dulse flakes for extra taste and saltiness. Pour over the burgers and enjoy!

# Desserts

Desserts are supposed to be a bit too much. Sometimes too fatty or to complex that can leave us spaced out for hours. One of my favourite desserts is ripe and delicious watermelon or durian, if fresh. But when you want to indulge yourself in something heartier, you can get inspired by unhealthy staples and create dairy-free ice cream, chocolate fudge or fruit jam for example.

## Ice cream

- 2 ripe, peeled and frozen bananas
- ½ cup of frozen blueberries or raspberries (or other frozen fruit of your choice)

Chop the banana in smaller pieces. Using Omega juicer with a blank tray make a banana whip with your frozen fruits. If you do not have the Omega juicer, use food processor with a bit of water. Process all ingredients until creamy. Transfer ice cream to a bowl, sprinkle with some fresh fruit or raisins and enjoy!

# Chocolate fudge tarts

For the tart base:

- ½ cup of raw almonds (soaked overnight)
- a small piece of banana (about 3 cm or 1 inch)

Take wet nuts and process in a food processor into very small chunks. Then add a piece of banana and let it mix well. Using wet hands divide your tart base into 4 small tart forms or 4 cupcake papers and form tart bottom.

For the filling:

- 4-5 Medjool dates or a cup of raisins
- the rest of banana
- 1 tablespoon of water (optional)

- ¼ of a teaspoon of vanilla beans
- 2 tablespoons of carob powder *(healthy replacement of cacao powder)*

In a food processor mix all dates (or raisins) until they start to bulk in a smooth paste (usually after about a minute). Add the rest of ingredients and process another minute or so, until all ingredients are well combined. Then put your filling onto your tart bases. You can leave it in a fridge for about half an hour to make it firmer or eat immediately. Decorate with fresh fruit like raspberry or blueberry and enjoy.

# Fruit jam

For the orange jam you will need:

- 3 tablespoons of chia seeds
- 2 Medjool dates or ¼ cup of raisins
- 3 medium oranges (peeled)

In a food processor mix oranges with dates until well combined, then pour it to a bowl and add chia seeds. Mix it well with a spoon and leave to rest for 15 minutes. Within that time you can mix it occasionally to check the consistency, as the chia seeds expand bringing it all to a yummy jam. For thicker jam add more chia seeds.

Try with a cup of blueberries, strawberries or raspberries instead of oranges for other jam flavours. Add vanilla beans or lemon juice for extra taste and aroma if you want to experiment more.

Chia seeds are extremely hydrating and have lots of health benefits. With no taste at all and gel-like consistency when mixed with any liquid, can be used in a colourful drinks, dressings and desserts, adding interesting texture with interesting visual effect.

# Herbs, spices and seaweed

Most herbs and spices are irritants, use them sparingly. When you give your body something that irritates it, the body will produce mucus to cover the irritant and push it through fast. But if it couldn't push it out quick enough, mucus cumulates in our tissues, for example—filling our sinus and making breathing more difficult. What's that in the corners of your eyes in the morning? It's mucus, with a bit of unwanted salt.

## About salt

Salt for example, is being given away through the skin with the perspiration (our sweat tastes salty). If our body needed that salt, why is it giving it away instead of holding on to it? If you go for a three days water fast, during that time your body will pull salt out of your skin through the liver, and you would give all the salt out through the liver. And then after if you start eating again but with no salt, and then you start to perspire, the sweat wouldn't be salty anymore, because there's nothing to kick out any more.

## Seaweed

I used to be a big fan of all seaweed, nori wraps and an algae salad were one of my favorites. Then I started to think, yes, we have all those life-giving minerals there, but what about all the toxic waste that's been dumped into the ocean? How about the catastrophes that happened in the past (by accident I'm sure), and ships licking out from their bellies with radioactive chemicals straight into the ocean. Sure the concentration levels are not that high to kill you immediately, but even if there's a tiny drop of arsenic in a bottle of water, I wouldn't drink it. Have we been so blind to

66

think it's not mixing everywhere? How about the observed marine mutations, the new colonies called nuclear plants? I wonder where did they get the name from? So no, I do not recommend eating seaweed from the ocean, no matter how organic it says it is. I just don't buy it.

# Fasting

Fasting is the best way to go while healing process starts. Whether it's a sickness or healing, our bodies will go better off without wasting the energy on digestion. When the fever kicks in or you are in pain, the best you can do is to trust your body; it knows what its doing and stay out of its way. Drink fresh water though. The healing process will go faster if you don't interfere, or interrupt it with a chicken soup or kebab. In the worst case scenario, your body will stop the cleaning and will wait for another, better time to continue when it has enough stored energy.

You can also do a prolonged fasting to let your body focus on healing, without waiting for an infection or a healing crisis. Before you do however, it is important to prepare your body and never do it without supervision. It is not so uncommon that people die after just 3 or 5 days of fasting, due to the flood of toxins kicking out as the body is not ready (it doesn't have enough energy or alkaline material, or it's too toxic) to manage it. Be aware of that!

If you are at age of 35 or more, and you've been eating a very bad diet all your life, chances are your body is very toxic. You may need a year of adding more fresh fruit and vegetables to your diet, while reducing toxic foods, to prepare yourself for 5-10 days of fasting. From my experience, I did a year of a raw food diet only, before I did my 11-days water fast and I had a very good experience. I was very week every third day, and quite vigorous, as you can be when just on water, every fourth and fifth day. I felt like I could continue the fast for another 10 days. I stopped though. That was the first time and I didn't want to take any chances.

See, we need to respect our bodies' conditions and where we are coming from, what diet and what health issues we've developed over the life time. By improving small things day by day our bodies will slowly get ready to clean themselves and you will get sick, probably reliving half of your past infections (see **Reactivation**, page 54), then start fasting, trusting your body knows what it's doing. It will be.

Other than that I recommend going to sleep with an almost empty stomach, meaning your last meal should be not later than three hours before going to bed. Then you will fast through the night. But if you ate just before a sleep time, fast in the morning. Give yourself 10-12 hours break before your next meal, or until you feel you are really hungry, but do not start your day with breakfast just because it's morning time. Listen to your body's needs instead. Fast until you feel a real hunger, then eat. It takes some discipline in the beginning but soon it becomes your new habit—it's that easy.

## Slow metabolism myth

Do not worry about the myth that your metabolism slowing down while fasting, it only slows down (and after 2-3 days it shuts down) the digestion. If you do a prolonged fasting from three days up, your body will switch normal digestive processes around at the end of the second day. And that's great, that's what we are looking for—we want all the energy to be focused on cleaning the house and healing.

But what if you do not eat your breakfast after waking up, as they recommend in all women's magazines? Well, nothing will happen. You will learn how to listen to your body's needs instead of a stranger telling you when you need to put the food in your body. Makes sense, does it? I also like the phrase my friend told me once—"You need to earn your breakfast. Wake up earlier and exercise!" That, my friend, will speed up your metabolism for sure, if you still worry about it.

# About digestion

## Digestion is distracting

Digestion is the second most absorbing and exhausting process in our body (first would be having a climax!). That's why we like numbing ourselves with food during tough times—problems fade away as we can't focus on them no more, busy with digestion. But our troubles can't be solved inside the stomach, you know it, but surely it's nice to forget.

You don't believe me? Test it! When upset, rate your state on a scale from 1 to 10, 10 being the most upset. Then have a piece of chocolate cake and tell me how did it change? If you feel bad about eating the cake now, that's a different problem already.

We are creatures of **habit**, and in this case, we conditioned ourselves to reach for a treat because it brings pleasure. But please be careful here—it is not the pleasure of eating delicious food you get, as crazy as it sounds, it's the numbing effect you linked to it you look for! Your problems become more distant and less stressful and our mind loves it. It's our primal survival mechanism to do whatever we can to keep away the suffering, you see? That is a main reason why we do not want to change our diet, even if the food we eat is killing us. Because stress is also deadly we, habit-controlled creatures, surrender to a blissful numbness, until one day we wake up and make amends.

## Being a lazy boss

Digestion starts in our mouth, when with teeth and saliva we break the food down. It's important to chew your food well, to make it ready for the next phase in our stomach but also to "let your body know" what is coming. This time is used to:

- **recognize** what chemical mixture your body has to create, to pair with the food in order to subtract the nutrients and transport them to cells,
- **what's missing,** in order to process the food and reach for the body's reserves,

- and **if toxins** are coming, to be ready rev up the metabolism (more energy will be needed) to process them out.

Not chewing your food is being a lazy boss, who puts all the work on others, expecting good results fast, without giving them even a notice what's coming up! You wouldn't like being treated like that at work, so why not to be gentle to your body, it's your home after all.

# Have a chemical cocktail to start with

When food reaches your stomach a dedicated chemical cocktail is created in order for it to be processed in our stomach. The more the food is processed, the more complex the digestion process and chemical mix are to deal with.

*Now imagine your stomach is a country border where every component will closely investigated for its "passport" and some will be paired with a "guard" (vitamins, minerals or enzymes) to be transported to body cells, without which nutrients can't be further processed and used. If we eat junk food it won't have the "passport" anymore and there will be troubles at the border, causing your body to negotiate and lose its resources. No one wants troubles on the border so always try to eat as much of alkaline foods as you can.*

## In order to process junk food the body will have to:

- **reach for its own reserves** to process the food (coming from the bones and other tissues to manufacture a "passport," it takes extra energy),
- produce **mucus** to cover irritating spices (it takes extra energy),
- prepare and treat the food with a **complex chemical mixture** to break it down (remember, the more processed the more complex and energy-consuming process) for the next part of the journey,
- expel **toxins** out, or if impossible—store them inside the body.

# After the party ends

After the horrendous effort your body made to process junk food in the stomach using its own reserves, it all travels to the intestines. Here dehydrated junk food will travel very slowly, sometimes for a couple of days before being expelled. The food that wasn't designed to stay in that long will start putrefying and as a result we experience often painful, smelly gas.

As the food travels through our intestines, some nutrients are being processed but if you eat a high-gluten diet (lots of whole wheat bread and pastas), your intestines will be covered with a glue-like substance, preventing any nutrients from being absorbed.

# Everything takes energy

Every process in your body requires energy, there's nothing for free. Eating foods without processing, chemical additives and spices, in its natural form, is the fastest and cheapest energy-wise for our bodies to process and save more for the cleansing processes. Ripe fruits and veggies, soaked nuts and sprouted seeds take little effort for our bodies to process and utilize it, without creating any nutritional deficiencies.

*Remember, if you'd eat a watermelon or large salad with some avocados, lettuce, tomatoes and cucumbers, in a healthy body the food will be processed within 2-4 hours.*

*If you eat a steak, to remove it with all the toxins as a side effect created in our body while processing it, it will take up to 3 days of eating just fruits and vegetables! What happens if you eat a steak with chips every day? Think about how much of it you've been carrying in your intestines for years!*

# Social situations

Here's an interesting aspect of us getting healthy, while everyone else is still an ignorant about their diet. How do we live with our families and friends on good terms, while pursuing our goal of getting healthy, by changing our diet so drastically?

I find it interesting that when I mention I am a vegan, everyone around becomes a nutrition specialist, suggesting that I'm not getting the nutrients from my food. Interestingly, most if not all of them, haven't had a real food for years!

I stopped answering those questions, because I do not feel like I need to explain myself or convince anybody, why should I? I wouldn't recommend lecturing or preaching either. Not only is it exhausting, but most of the time, not very welcome.

Instead I just do what I feel is right for me at the time, knowing what I know and I stick to it as long as it work. If you find yourself in a situation you crave some of the junk foods, go ahead and have some, just be aware that you can get sick the next day, as your body will try to expel toxins vigorously. The healthier you get the more rapid this process will be.

If you know you are going for a barbecue with your friends or to a restaurant you can do few things:

- eat before so you are not hungry, it's easier to stay away from the junk food you still have cravings for,
- prepare your meal to take with you, make some more so you could share with others, especially if it's a fancy recipe, so they can see, a raw food diet is not just a lettuce and carrot,
- have integrity and do not argue with others, it will save you a lot of energy,
- pain this picture in your head: in 10, 15 years your friends will be asking you advice what to do to look so young and be healthy. Mark my words!

# Be brave! Be healthy! Be beautiful!

# Relationship with food

Think about the food and your relationship with it. What does it mean to you, being in relationship? Do you love your food so much you can't say goodbye to some junk food? Is it a toxic relationship? How about being in a loving relationship, with foods that love you back? Think about wanting that kind of relationship with food, and transformation into health will be easier and much more rewarding.

# Shortly about bulimia

For those who do not know, bulimia is a dangerous eating disorder that may lead to death. The problem with bulimics is that they can't stop obsessing about food. The food is always in their mind and they can't control the need for eating, and most of the time they chose to binge on junk food they wouldn't normally eat.

Some bulimic can easily eat a 3 kg (close to 6 lbs) bag of French fries during one sitting, to give you an idea, or eat 10-12 times a day, purging shortly after each meal, and after all that, going to sleep hungry. That is my experience at least.

Bulimia is not a joke and it kills slowly. Some of the dangers a bulimic has to face is cardiac arrest, ketoacidosis, gastric rupture, low blood pressure or hypotension, seizures, electrolyte imbalance and malnutrition, stomach and gullet pain, depression and often social alienation. It can also eventually lead to a slow weight gain, as the stomach is getting more and more stressed and it can't get empty through purging any more. One of the scariest images that tortured me along with the chains of bulimia itself was the idea of my stomach breaking and a sudden death. Even though, when the crisis was over, I continued binging and purging over and over. Sadly, I couldn't stop this addiction.

Now, once you understand that it is an addiction you may wonder, if there's a structural program or therapy that can help? Yes there is, not one but many, but it never worked for me. Like with every addiction there need to be a way to replace your addiction with something, at least for a short while, long enough to distract yourself. What I discovered after the years of torture was eating the right kind of foods in abundance helps! I started stuffing myself with fruit that was the only thing I had to focus on. I still could binge, but fruit has never led me to purging. Ever! I knew this food won't make me sick or fat, as long as I will eat just that, ideally just one kind of fruit at the time. I felt so satisfied and happy with what was inside my body, I knew it will heal and nourish me, so I never felt the need for purging.

Understand this, the food didn't heal me from bulimia, but it gave me an ease, a rest I needed to recover from never-ending cycle. Se, even though I knew I was killing myself, I simply couldn't just stop. Only when I started eating juicy and sweet fruit meals and lots of greens in my gigantic salads, I started getting back to life and back in control with my eating habits. I did it on my own, without any bulimic specialist or group support. I didn't know I was strong enough to break the habit, but it was easier than I though.

Of course there were dangerous turns on my way and I failed a few times. But every time I learned something valuable and I came up with a list of what to do to survive.

## My survival list

- always have fruit at home
- do shopping when full
- never go out hungry
- when going out always have dry fruit with you (my favorite – dates! I was eating 2 kg a day in the first month of going raw! I was so anemic and I was so happy I could eat something sweet without feeling guilty I was eating them every time I craved sweetness and always in abundance!)
- when you crave sweetness – eat your sweet fruit, dry or fresh in abundance
- when you crave sour or salty – you need minerals coming from greens and veggies, therefore eat some celery or a salad with tomatoes and avocado with good amount of lemon juice (use a lot of lemons, you won't need salt)

I know now I have failed if I break one of the above rules, so I follow them not to let myself down anymore. Now I let myself to occasionally go out and eat something cooked knowing it's not the best food of all, but there's no more guilt, because I always make sure to eat a large salad with it or before, to bring the alkaline to my body and balance my meal.

If you want to know more about my way to recovery from bulimia through the transition diet, or you have questions please write to me at hello@fruitarianna.com. I'd be grateful for the opportunity to help anybody with this dreadful condition that made me a slave of food for so long.

In the beginning of 2014 look my new book—*Bulimia without therapy. Welcome to the world of fruit*, will available on Amazon, createspace, sweetvegannature.com and fruit-powered.com.

# Food combinations

Proper food combining assures the best results for fast digestion and optimal nutrition. Different foods require different digestive enzymes while processed in our stomach, and if you bad, they may cancel each other, resulting in longer digestion and putrefying food, and sometimes a stomachache. Apply those simple rules of the proper food combining and you will get the best of your food.

The chart on the next page may seem overwhelming but if you remember not to eat melons with other food, keep bananas away from oranges and never eat fruit with veggies, especially fatty ones, than you should be just fine. In time you'll develop sensitivity that will guide you without any doubts.

# Food Combining Chart

## DO NOT EAT FRUIT WITH ANY OTHER FOOD EXCEPT GREEN NON-STARCHY VEGETABLES

### ACID FRUIT
Blackberries   Pineapple
Grapefruit   Raspberries
Lemon   Strawberries
Lime   Tangerines
Orange   Tomatoes[1]

[Eat before other fruits]

### SUB-ACID FRUIT
Apple   Kiwi
Apricot   Mango
Blueberries   Nectarine
Cherimoya   Papaya
Cherries   Peach
Fresh Fig   Pear
Grapes   Plums

### SWEET FRUIT
Bananas
Dates
Dried Fruit
Thompson &
Muscat Grapes
Persimmon
Raisins

### MELON
Cantaloupe   Honey Dew
Casaba   Persian
Crane   Sharlyn
Crenshaw   Watermelon

[Eat before other fruits]

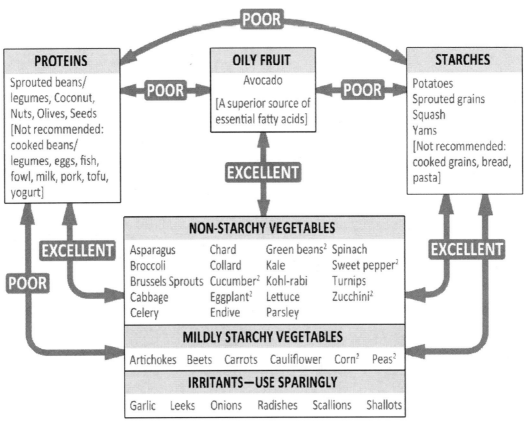

**PROTEINS**

Sprouted beans/
legumes, Coconut,
Nuts, Olives, Seeds
[Not recommended:
cooked beans/
legumes, eggs, fish,
fowl, milk, pork, tofu,
yogurt]

**OILY FRUIT**

Avocado

[A superior source of
essential fatty acids]

**STARCHES**

Potatoes
Sprouted grains
Squash
Yams
[Not recommended:
cooked grains, bread,
pasta]

POOR · POOR · POOR · POOR · EXCELLENT · EXCELLENT · EXCELLENT

**NON-STARCHY VEGETABLES**

Asparagus   Chard   Green beans[2]   Spinach
Broccoli   Collard   Kale   Sweet pepper[2]
Brussels Sprouts   Cucumber[2]   Kohl-rabi   Turnips
Cabbage   Eggplant[2]   Lettuce   Zucchini[2]
Celery   Endive   Parsley

**MILDLY STARCHY VEGETABLES**

Artichokes   Beets   Carrots   Cauliflower   Corn[2]   Peas[2]

**IRRITANTS—USE SPARINGLY**

Garlic   Leeks   Onions   Radishes   Scallions   Shallots

[1] Tomatoes only combine with non-starchy vegetables, seeds, nuts, olives, avocados, cucumbers and sweet peppers.

[2] Botanically classified as a fruit, but its bio-chemical composition places it in a non-fruit food combining category.

*Special thanks to Dr. David Klein, founder of the Colitis & Crohn's Health Recovery Center and publisher and executive editor of Vibrance magazine, for sharing the chart.*

# Alkaline foods index

## Extremely alkaline

Cantaloupe, celery, dates, figs (dried), grapes, kiwi, lemons, limes, mango, melons, papaya, parsley, passion fruit, pears, pineapple, raisins, watercress, watermelon.

## Moderately alkaline

Apples, apple cider vinegar, alfalfa sprouts, apricots, avocados, bananas (ripe), beets, bell peppers, broccoli, cabbage, carob, cauliflower, currants, figs (fresh), ginger (fresh), grapes (less sweet and sour), grapefruit, guavas, herbs (leafy green), lettuce (leafy green), nectarine, oranges, peaches, pears (less sweet), peas (fresh, sweet), pumpkin (sweet), raspberries, strawberries, squash, sweet corn (fresh), turnip.

## Slightly alkaline

Almonds, artichokes (jerusalem), Brussels sprouts, cherries, coconut (fresh), cucumbers, eggplant, leek, mushrooms, okra, olives (ripe), onions, radishes, tomatoes (sweet).

# About veganism[11]

Veganism is not defined as a diet, but a way of living. While vegans follow an animal-free diet, they also do not wear animals or use them for entertainment or any other purpose.

## Moral schizophrenia

If it is wrong to act violently to a dog or cat just for enjoyment or convenience, how can we justify the horrible things we do to other animals? We certainly do not need to eat animal products to be healthy; we do so only because it is a habit and we enjoy the taste of these products. Some of us try to address this inconsistency by purchasing products that are marketed as "humane" or as produced "ethically." However, as you'll see, these words are meaningless and actually do very little to give animals a better life. In any case, these terms encourage the public to believe it is okay to exploit animals simply because we enjoy it. This strange contradiction is our "moral schizophrenia." We can overcome this social affliction and respect life by going vegan.

### Can't we just consume "humane" animal products?

Asking how "well" we should treat animals is the wrong question in the first place. Supposed "happy" animals are really treated no differently than those in factory farms. For example, there are no special transport vehicles for "humanely-raised" animals. The process of transport is the same as conventional animals and is a miserable, often fatal experience. Animals are forced onto trucks with weapons, prods, and even forklifts. Inside, it doesn't matter if the animals are terrified or in pain, as long as they get to the slaughterhouse alive.

> "As with any other form of industrialized animal use, consumers have the choice either to participate in it or to refuse the products of exploitation and opt out of the demand-supply cycle altogether. (...)

---

[11] Inspired by and quoted after the Vegan Starter Kit (see: SweetVeganNature.com/vegan-starter-kit/)

*Humans have no need for animal products, and the increasing number of vegans on the planet is a testament to how easy it is to live a healthy, fulfilling life without participating in the systematic abuse and unnecessary killing that goes on in the animal industry every day.*

*— Angel Flinn*

Animals suffer from cold, hunger, thirst, untreated infections, and illnesses during transport. This is not, however, a matter of irresponsible slaughterhouse workers. As long as these animals are objects of property, they cannot have rights. To some, "humane" legislation appears to get us closer to having better lives for animals.

Animal welfare legislation calls for larger confinements and methods of slaughter which supposedly cause less pain. However, these reforms are industry practices which do away with economically wasteful and outdated practices. Animal welfare fosters more economically beneficial standards for producers and makes the public feel better about exploiting animals through marketing.

It's not about "them," the producers, it's about us. We are the consumers, we are the ones paying for this practice to happen. The first, most important thing we can do to address this violence is to go vegan.

*[The use of humane slaughter methods] ... results in safer and better working conditions... brings about the improvement of products and economies in slaughtering operations; and produces other benefits for producers, processors, and consumers which tend to expedite an orderly flow of livestock and livestock products...*

*— United States Humane Methods of Slaughter Act*

(Notice the lack of any mention of an animal's wellbeing. Welfarism is about using animals efficiently and cost-effectively.) It's better for your health (animal foods cause physical harm); it's better for the environment (animal agriculture is an ecological disaster); and, most importantly, it's the morally right thing to do.

# Is veganism good for the planet?

*"About 2,000 pounds of grains must be supplied to livestock in order to produce enough meat and other livestock products to support a person for a year,*

*whereas 400 pounds of grain eaten directly will support a person for a year. Thus, a given quantity of grain eaten directly will feed 5 times as many people as it will if it is eaten indirectly by humans in the form of livestock products...."*

— *M.E. Ensminger, PhD*

Consuming a plant-based diet also has significant benefits for our environment. For example, the amount of potatoes we can produce from an acre of land is about 40,000 lbs compared to only 250 lbs of cow flesh supported from the same acre. When we feed plants to animals in order to eat the animal, we waste an enormous amount of food. For only one pound of cow flesh, 16 lbs of plant food and 5,000 gallons of water are required.

Compare that to 25 gallons of water for a pound of wheat. Animal agriculture is also responsible for most of the food-borne illness epidemics from water runoff. Our use of animals contributes significantly to greenhouse gas emissions as well as the destruction of forests for grazing. More than 250 million acres of forests are cleared every year in the US alone for this purpose.

# Is veganism sustainable?

Considering the amount of waste produced by animal agriculture, it's staggering to think how much plant-based food could potentially be grown using the same resources used for animals. Essentially, we have to feed animals plant foods constantly as they mature. After three to four years of harvesting and cycling this plant food through an animal, the animal is killed and eaten just once. Imagine instead, each of those four years was used to grow plant food to be directly consumed by humans.

# What's wrong with milk?

## Health aspect

Somewhere along the way, humanity decided that cow's milk is just good for us and we started treating kids with it! Since 1900 our consumption of dairy products increased by 600% and it doesn't seem to stop there for long. "A glass of milk a day will keep the doctor away!" or was it supposed to be an apple? Who changed that for us?

Cow's milk was designed to make its baby to grow during the first year about half pound a day! If you really care about that weight-gaining supplement, by all means—eat more cheese.

The truth is, no other species drinks milk of another species, and that's weird we do. Cow's milk is incompatible with our bodies and it has nothing to offer to humans. Inside our bodies it becomes acid producing and as an effect, it robs us of precious nutrients, while we try to neutralize and digest dairy product. On top of that, milk contains many things you don't want to see there (see the picture below).

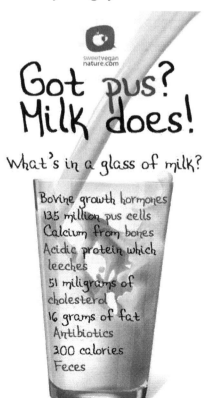

In spite of all the studies made, giving proof that drinking cow's milk is harmful to our bodies, why is it still so hard to believe for many.

We drink milk only out of habit or, rather, because of the addiction to **casomorphin**, a powerful opiate, designed by nature to keep a calf close to its mother.

*"The most wholesome cow's milk from organically raised bovines naturally contains a powerful opiate in the morphine family called casomorphin. Concentrated milk products (cheese, ice cream and milk chocolate) contain concentrated quantities of these addictive narcotics."*

—*source: NotMilk.com*

If you think you can never give up cheese you have a similar problem to that of a junkie drug addict. Now you know the truth, the decision what you are going to do is yours.

Maybe you decide to explore plant-based alternatives made of almonds, cashews, oats or soy? The only think you give up is animal product full of antibiotics, hormones, cholesterol and pus. What you gain is freedom from addiction and drugs which just make your head cloudy and rob you of health.

## Moral aspect

Aside from the health aspect of drinking milk and eating cheese it's important to understand that dairy is not a cruelty-free product at all, as many think. During his the most famous lecture Gary Yourofsky painted this picture, that changed lives of hundreds people. Maybe it will move you as it did move me.

> *"If we agree that a cow, and any other animal for that matter, has eyes to see, a nose to breathe through, ears to listen to with, a heart to pump blood and a brain to think, how can anyone believe the cow doesn't have feelings? Do you think that she doesn't have any connection with her baby? That she enjoys life in an unnatural setting such as a factory farm, being raped repeatedly to be able to give birth to the calf that will never get the milk meant for it? That she won't live long enough because of the abuse and constant stress her body is going through? Consider that next time you think of a slice of cheese."*

I wanted to leave you with a few more quotations that may shock and inspire you. I wish you all the love and peace in your lifetime. May you never have to suffer like animals do for us.

> *"After repeated cycles of forced impregnations, painful births, relentless milking, and crushing bereavements, their spirit gives, their bodies wither, their milk dries up. At the age when, in nature, a female cow would barely enter adulthood, the life of a dairy cow is over. When her milk 'production' declines, she and her other 'spent' herd mates are trucked off to slaughter. Some are pregnant. All are still lactating. As they are shoved towards death, they drip milk onto the killing floor... All dairy operations, including Organic, exist solely by doing to millions of defenseless females the worst thing anyone can do to a mother. Dairy consumers support this practice with their purchases."*

> —*"Milk Comes from a Grieving Mother", leaflet by Peaceful Prairie Sanctuary*

Remember,

*"Veganism is not about giving anything up or losing anything; it is about gaining the peace within yourself that comes from embracing nonviolence and refusing to participate in the exploitation of the vulnerable."*

*—Gary L. Francione*

*"Go vegan. It's better for your health (animal foods cause physical harm); it's better for the environment (animal agriculture is an ecological disaster); and, most importantly, it's the morally right thing to do."*

*— Gary L. Francione*

*"...we have so many alternatives that don't involve using animals as our things. Using animal products is unnecessary, it harms animals, and it inevitably makes us responsible for the killing of a sentient being—whose life is the only life that being has—for transparently trivial reasons."*

*— Eric Prescott*

# Recommended media

## Websites

- *www.SweetVeganNature.com*
  Sweet Vegan Nature provides you with articles about food and health, losing weight and smart choices. Available programs for free and premium users will take you on a weekend detox or through the 30 days challenge. Find support on your transition to healthier choices.

- *www.Fruitarianna.com*
  Learn about nutrition and have fun reading a comic! Also vegan t-shirts and bags available.

- *www.Cronometer.com*
  CRON-O-Meter records nutrition and health data, including calories.

- *www.30BananasADay.com*
  The world's largest world's largest raw vegan social network, featuring a forum and videos, with more than 17,000 members as of spring 2013.

- *www.MeganElizabeth.com*
  Megan Elizabeth features videos—many quite long and informative—on raw food tips and recipes as well as healthful living.

- *www.FitOnRaw.com*
  Swayze Foster offers hundreds of videos on a low-fat, fruit-based diet. She serves up tips, recipes, news and views on the science behind raw food and much more.

- *www.Raw-Food-Health.net*
  Explore Andrew Perlot's scientifically valid explanations for why a fruit-based diet is best, raw food recipes, advice for getting and staying on the diet and more.

- ***www.TheFruitarian.com***
  Long-distance runner Michael Arnstein is one of the most extreme raw food runners there are. He shares his experiences regarding his performance improvement and incredibly fast body regeneration since he switched to a 100% raw food diet.

- ***www.Vitamix.com***
  Explore blenders made by Vitamix, the world leader in high-performance blending equipment.

# Books

- Visit the ***Fruit-Powered store*** for a growing selection of titles.

- ***The China Study***
  T. Colin Campbell brings the most comprehensive study of nutrition ever conducted and the startling implications for diet, weight loss, and long-term health. Available also in audiobook format.

- ***The 80/10/10 Diet***
  Doug Graham has taken the increasingly popular and tremendously successful low-fat, plant-based diet and turbo-charged it for unprecedented, off-the-charts results.

- ***Green for Life***
  Discover a wealth of information in Victoria Boutenko's book on green nutrition. It's ideal for anyone who wishes to develop a healthful diet.

# Films

- ***Fat, Sick & Nearly Dead***
  Overweight, reliant on steroids and suffering from an autoimmune disease, Joe Cross embarks on a juice fast across America. Along the way, he meets a 429-pound trucker who suffers from the same disease. This film chronicles their recoveries of health.

- *Forks Over Knives*

  *Forks Over Knives* examines the claim that most if not all the degenerative diseases that afflict us can be controlled or even reversed by rejecting animal-based and processed foods.

- *Food Matters*

  *Food Matters* sets about uncovering the trillion-dollar worldwide "sickness industry" and gives people some scientifically verifiable solutions for overcoming illness naturally.

- *Healing Cancer From Inside Out*

  This film focuses on the failings of conventional cancer treatments and shows how cancer can be successfully healed with dietary treatments and natural supplementation and includes interviews with people who have reversed cancers using diet.

- **The Best Vegan Speech by Gary Yourofsky**

  The lecture that changed life of thousands! The best lecture about why being vegan ever recorded (http://www.sweetvegannature.com/the-best-vegan-speach-by-gary-yourofsky/).

- **Other vegan movies compilation**

  Watch movies here http://www.sweetvegannature.com/vegan-movies/ (e.g. *Earthlings*).

## Magazine

- *www.Fruit-Powered.com – Raw Food Magazine*

  Brian Rossiter uses his journalist's eye to track success stories, tips and guides on how to succeed on a raw food diet. Together with his guest writers he shines a light on a nutrition science that can be confusing sometimes. Brian also collects the best of the recipes and books from the raw food world, so check out his growing vibrant magazine.

- ***Vibrance***

  An independent magazine published and edited by <u>Dr. David Klein</u>, *Vibrance* promotes healthful, essential and ecologically positive products and services, as per the "healthful living" lifestyle tenets taught by Natural Hygiene. Its website also offers a first-rate bookstore and much more.


# Podcast

- ***Raw Food Health Podcast***

  <u>Andrew Perlot</u>'s podcast is designed to help one improve his or her health, vitality and fitness through the adoption of a low-fat raw vegan diet.

Made in the USA
Middletown, DE
17 March 2017